PeriAnesthesia

101

For Nurses

The reference guide for nurses
working in the pre-operative
and post-operative units.

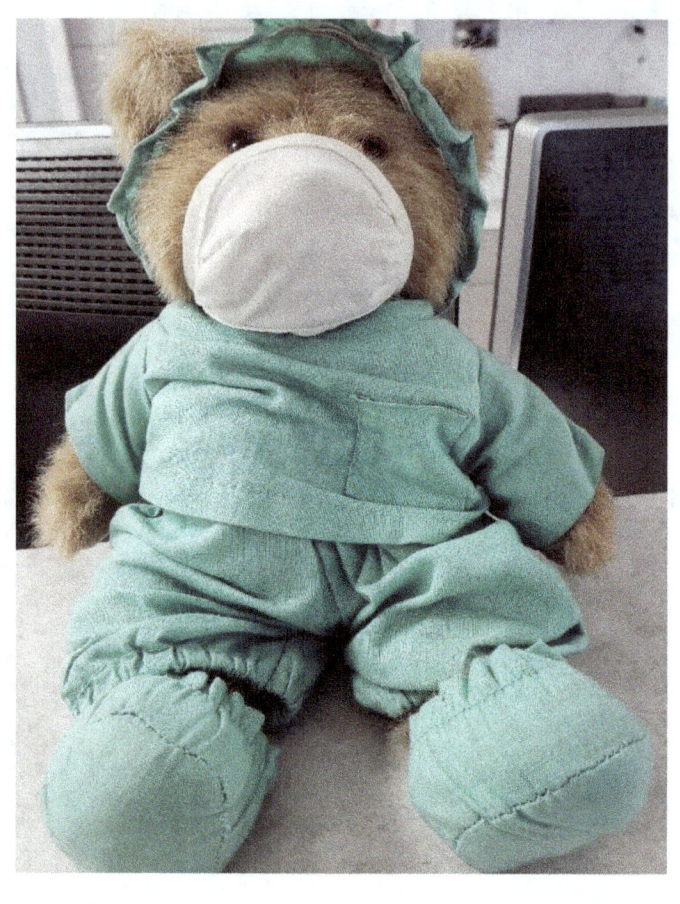

Contents

5

PeriAnesthesia 101 for Nurses Introduction

Welcome to PeriAnesthesia 101 for Nurses! This book was written for nurses who work in the Pre-operative and post-operative surgical areas. Perianesthesia nursing encompasses preadmission, day of surgery preparation, post-anesthesia phases 1 and 2, and extended observation. You may be a nurse who gets a patient ready for surgery or is there to help the patient wake up. Perianesthesia nurses work in hospitals, outpatient surgery centers, and outpatient offices.

This book was written for nurses who may be new to the profession, need study material for a certification test, or want a handy reference guide. This book contains information on how to care for patients undergoing different types of surgery, including pre-op and post-op care. There is a section on abbreviations, a glossary, a large section on medications, and a section on general nursing care which will discuss different types of scoring tools, lab values, the culture of safety, and legal issues.

There are in-depth sections on each surgery specialty, including ortho, urology, gynecology, neurology, and others.

Certification

This book is a resource for nurses who wish to sit for the CAPA (Certified Ambulatory Perianesthesia Nurse) and the CPAN (Certified Post Anesthesia Nurse). In this book, you will find chapters specific to body systems and situations you will see as a nurse in the PeriAnesthesia world. At the end of the book, you will find practice questions for both the CAPA and the CPAN with answers and rationales.

The Certified ambulatory Peri Anesthesia Nurse, or CAPA, is for nurses with at least 1,200 hours of direct patient care experience in pre-anesthesia, phase 2, day of surgery procedures, or extended care of post-anesthesia patients.

The Certified Post Anesthesia Nurse, or CPAN, is for nurses with at least 1,200 hours of direct patient care in the phase 1 recovery room.

The CAPA and CPAN certification exams are designed by the American Board of Perianestesia Nursing Certification (ABPANC). Please visit cpancapa.org to read the certification candidate handbook for details on testing and for other study help.

For those nurses planning on taking the CAPA, CPAN, or both exams, read the exam blueprint found online to help determine areas of strength and areas that demonstrate an opportunity for learning. Your facility may not perform a large variety of surgeries, so you may wish to study those that are unfamiliar to you. Design a study plan that is set in a reasonable time frame to learn and review the material. Ask your co-workers and friends that are PeriAnesthesia nurses if they have study materials to share. Determine if a study group would benefit you and see if anyone is interested. A benefit of a study group is the moral support that can be provided by others undertaking the same adventure.

After deciding on a test date, ask your employer if there are funds available to help with the test cost or study materials. Some facilities pay a certification premium for nurses who are certified. Once you pass your exam, don't forget to tell your employer to get that sweet certification money!

Many people suffer from test anxiety, this is normal. To help you feel better, before the day of the exam, make sure you know where the testing location is. If the testing location is far from home, leave a little early to avoid more anxiety if there is traffic or if you get lost. Wear comfortable clothing. You may be asked to roll up your sleeves and roll down your socks to check for contraband. If you are taking a test at home where the online proctor needs to see the whole room you are in, make sure your camera is ready. At the testing center, read all instructions. There may be ways to mark your answers to go back or the ability to skip a question for later. To help you not get overstimulated by all the answers, read the question, answer it in your head, and then look at the answers. If your answer is there, it is probably the right one.

After you pass your test, celebrate! Becoming certified is a huge achievement! You will remain certified for three years. After three years, you will need to enter the credits and points you earned to recertify, or you can retake the test. For most nurses, one test is enough.

To recertify, you will go onto the ABPANC website and enter your points and credits. I recommend doing this throughout the three years, so you don't forget anything.

In 1863 Florence Nightingale used separate rooms for patients recovering from anesthesia

Abbreviations

- AACN- American Association of Colleges of Nursing

- ABPANC- American Board of

- Perianesthesia Nursing Certification

- AORN- Association of Perioperative Registered Nurses

- ACLS- Advanced Cardiac Life Support

- AE- Adverse Event

- ASPAN- The American Society of PeriAnesthesia Nurses

- ASU- Ambulatory Surgery Unit

- BPD- borderline personality disorder

- CRNA- Certified Registered Nurses Anesthetist

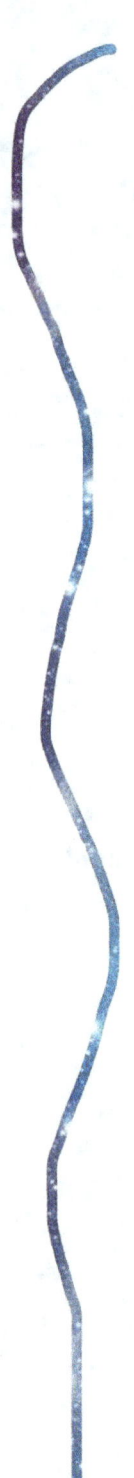

- ECT- Electroconvulsive Therapy- This is a therapy for patients with a diagnosis of depression.

- FBS- Fasting Blood Sugar

- HIPPA- Health Insurance Portability and Accountability Act. Protects sensitive patient information.

- MAC- Monitored anesthesia care.

- MAOI- Monoamine Oxidase Inhibitor

- MH- Mental Health

- OSA- Obstructive Sleep Apnea

- PACU- Post-Anesthesia Care Unit

- PALS- Pediatric Advanced Life Support

- PONV- Post-Op Nausea and Vomiting

- RICE- Rest, Ice, Compression, Elevation

Glossary

- Acidosis- This leads to an increased hydrogen ion concentration in the blood.

- Apneustic breathing- Breathing that demonstrates prolonged inspiration.

- Allodynia pain- Caused by a stimulus that does not normally cause pain.

- Arthrodesis- Fusion or immobilization of a joint.

- Chlorhexidine gluconate (CHG)- Antibacterial agent effective against a wide variety of organisms. Used to prep patients for surgery. Patients may need to take a CHG shower the night before surgery at their home. The patient may be wiped down with CHG-impregnated wipes before surgery to help prevent infection.

- Colonization- Microorganisms in an area that do not cause disease.

- Droplet transmission- Airborne droplets of microorganisms that can travel 0 to 3 feet.

- Dysesthesia- An unpleasant, abnormal sensation.

- Endoscopy- Visual exam with an endoscope. Procedures may be through a natural orifice such as the mouth, anus, cervix, or urethra. An endoscopic procedure may also be completed through a small incision with the use of a trocar.

- Hypercarbia- Increasing partial pressure of carbon dioxide (PaCO2), respiratory acidosis.

- Laparotomy- Incision of the abdominal wall, commonly used for exploration. The incision may be vertical or transverse. The patient will typically have a large abdominal wound. This type of surgery has been reduced with the introduction of laparoscopy, which only requires small incisions to place the instruments.

- MAC- Monitored anesthesia care. A type of anesthesia involves the patient being able to breathe on their own with the anesthesia provider standing by to assist as needed. This type of anesthesia may be called twilight anesthesia. The patient can relax for the procedure but does not need to be intubated.

- Malingering- A conscious exaggeration of an effect of a disease or condition. Older doctors and nurses may use this term.

- N95 respirator- a face mask that is 95% efficient at removing 0.3um particles and is not oil-resistant.

- Osteotomy- Incision into a bone.

- Tenotomy- Incision of a tendon.

General PeriAnesthesia care

- Pre-anesthesia phase. This area is focused on preparation for surgery. This is the pre-op area. Assessment of the patient's physical, mental, and spiritual needs is completed to identify issues needing to be addressed. If this phase is completed on the day of surgery, the nursing care may also include education on what to expect in the following phases of care and possibly discharge teaching. When nurses are proficient in this area of nursing, they demonstrate their knowledge by taking the CAPA exam.

  - Staffing for Pre-anesthesia depends on the patient's acuity, age of patients, and, if needed, sedation for pre-operative nerve blocks. If a nurse cares for a patient receiving conscious sedation, that nurse should have no other responsibilities.

- Post-anesthesia phase 1. This is the immediate post-operative area. This is the PACU or recovery room. The patient may need assistance with breathing or other life-saving measures. The patient requires constant attention.

Nurses who are proficient in this area can take the CPAN exam.

- o Staffing for phase 1 post-anesthesia care should be one nurse to one patient or one nurse to two patients. New admissions to the unit should be closely monitored until critical needs are met, such as airway and vital signs are stable, the initial assessment is completed, and the patient is calm, without combativeness or agitation.

- o There should be at least two nurses in the unit, one caring for the patient and one immediately available to assist as needed. One nurse in the unit must be competent in phase 1 nursing care.

- o The nurse may have two patients if both are hemodynamically stable, conscious, over age eight, or under age eight with a family or caregiver at the bedside.

- o The nurse may have one patient if under eight years old and unconscious.

- o The nurse may have one patient who is not conscious but hemodynamically stable, with a stable airway over the age of eight, and one patient who is conscious and stable.

- o Occasionally one patient who is critical and unstable may require two nurses.

- Post-anesthesia phase 2. The patients in this area are preparing to go home. This is the area where the patient receives discharge instructions. The patient still requires monitoring for complications related to surgery or medications. Nurses with this specialty can sit for the CAPA certification.

- o Staffing for phase 2 should be one nurse for up to three patients. Staffing decisions should be made based on patient safety.

- o The nurse can care for three patients if over the age of eight or under age eight with family present.

- o If the patient is under the age of eight and without family or support staff, the nurse-to-patient ratio should be one nurse to two patients.

- o Two staff members are required to be in the unit at all times. One must be an RN competent in phase 2 nursing.

- o Staffing will be one nurse to one patient if a patient becomes unstable and requires transfer to a higher level of care.

- o A patient may be what is termed "Fast-tracked." This occurs when a patient bypasses phase one recovery and is sent directly to phase two recovery. The patient is awake or easily arousable, on room air or at baseline, has minimal pain, and is hemodynamically stable.

- Extended care. This is an area where patients require extended observation after discharge from phase 2.

- o Staffing for extended care should be one nurse for three to five patients. These patients are typically awaiting transport home or being held due to waiting to be transported to an inpatient bed.

- o Two staff members should be in the unit at all times. One staff member is an RN competent in caring for the patient population.

- Blended Care. This environment involves the care of patients who belong in multiple phases of care. Clinical judgment is required to determine safe staffing levels. Patients in different levels of care may share the same physical space. An effort must be made to ensure the privacy and confidentiality of all patients.

Isolation precautions

- Airborne precautions- Measles, SARS, varicella-chicken pox, mycobacterium tuberculosis. Use a negative pressure room if available.

- Contact precautions- Clostridium difficile, norovirus, rotavirus.

- Droplet- Pertussis, influenza, diphtheria

    ERAS- Enhanced recovery after surgery- Reducing variance and improving efficiency in patient outcomes. This is practiced by all disciplines caring for the patient. You are following evidence-based best practices to give the patient the best outcome. The use of clinical pathways can help staff follow accepted practices.

Patient Education

Assessing the patient's preferred learning method will help the patient retain the information provided. Learning styles may include:

- Visual- Show the patients pictures or videos and provide written materials.

- Auditory- Patients that learn through hearing may prefer verbal instructions.

- Kinesthetic- Patients learn through physical activities. Allow these patients hands-on learning—for example, return demonstrations of new medical devices.

Assess learning needs and gaps in knowledge. Consider the patient's support system and who needs to share in the education. Determine if there are barriers to learning that may be cognitive, physical, language, or financial. Assess motivation and set realistic goals.

Legal Forms, Terms, and Orders

If the patient has a Do Not Resuscitate (DNR) order preoperatively, the surgeon will ask the patient if this continues throughout the perioperative process.

- Autonomy- The right to determine what happens to your body by deciding on treatments and types of care.

- A living will- the patient has made future healthcare decisions for themselves in the event they become incapacitated and cannot speak for themselves. It may be called an advance directive.

- A durable power of attorney- The patient has named someone to be their proxy in the event the patient cannot speak for themselves.

- Conscious objection- When a patient or family is making decisions that conflict with the nurse's values, such as abortion care, removing life-sustaining care, or refusal of blood products. The nurse may refuse to care for patients on the grounds that the care will cause the nurse moral distress. Refusal cannot be because of bias or convenience.

- AND- Allow natural death. Comfort measures only.

- POLST- A physician's order regarding life-sustaining treatment.

- PSDA- Patient Self Determination Act- The patient is legally required to receive information about advanced directives.

- State Nursing Boards define the nurses' scope of practice within the state.

- Malpractice

  - Failure to provide care that meets the required standard of care.

- An act of negligence or omission that deviates from the accepted level of care that harms a patient.

- Negligence

  - Duty exists between Parties.
  - Breach of duty.
  - Breach of duty is a cause of injury.
  - Injuries or harm occur.
  - Failure to provide care in a way a reasonable person would, failure to act in accordance with the standard of care.

- Assault- a threat or act that causes a person to fear injury or physical touch.

- Battery- Non-consensual touching of a person's body or extension of the body in an offensive or injurious manner. If CPR is performed in the hospital on a person with a DNR order, this is battery.

Informed consent- The surgeon explains the following:

- Diagnosis
- Procedure
- Risks
- Benefits
- Alternatives

When a nurse signs as a witness on a consent, the nurse only witnesses the signature, not that the patient fully understands.

➢ Implied consent- in emergency situations, consent may be legally presumed when the patient cannot speak for themselves.

For a patient having surgery with bilateral body parts, such as the arm or leg, the surgeon will mark with a special marker the side they will perform surgery on. This helps prevent wrong-site surgeries, which are never events- never should happen. The patient should be awake and aware when the surgeon marks the area so the patient can agree.

Children are considered emancipated minors when married, have a child of their own, or are in the military. These patients are no longer reliant on parental control.

Abuse and Neglect

Nurses are mandated reporters. Signs and symptoms of abuse and neglect for vulnerable patients should be reported to the appropriate authorities. Follow your facility's policy on how to report. Fines and jail time may be imposed on nurses who fail to report.

Signs and symptoms of abuse may include:

- Bite marks
- Bruises in the groin or genitals
- Bruises in hidden areas
- Fractured teeth, bruises around the face or head
- Thermal injuries

- Lethargy, poor feeding, and retinal hemorrhage- may be shaken baby syndrome.
- Spiral fractures, rib fractures
- Frequent urinary tract infections from sexual abuse
- Signs of neglect
- Developmental delays in otherwise healthy children.

The American Nurses Association published the *Code of Ethics* in 1950

Evidence-based practice

- Assists with clinical decision-making using a problem-solving approach.
- Analysis of research
- Nursing and other clinical expertise
- Best evidence

- The goal is to improve patient outcomes, provide quality, cost-effective care, and reduce variations in practice.
- There are three levels of evidence when preparing recommendations.

  - A- Multiple randomized trials
  - B- Single randomized trials or nonrandomized trials
  - C-Expert opinions, case studies

➤ Quality/ Process Improvement
  - Plan – Do – Check – Act, or Plan -Do- Study- Act- A continuous cycle, a change model.

NPO guidelines:

2 hours clear liquids
4 hours for breast milk
6 hours for infant formula
6 hours for nonhuman milk
6 hours light meal.

Guidelines are just that. If the patient has recently eaten, ask the surgeon and the anesthesia provider. The patient may not be able to wait for surgery due to the patient's condition.

Gum and hard candy can cause increased stomach secretions. If the patient chews gum before the surgery, the anesthesia provider may cancel or delay surgery.

As great as smoking cigarettes is, smoking within eight hours of surgery is probably not a good idea. Smoking can increase the amount of carbon monoxide in the blood, increase airway irritation, decrease oxygenation during anesthesia, and increase gastric volume.

Culture of Safety

Tenets of a safety culture:
Communication
Advocacy
Competency
Efficiency
Teamwork

A culture of safety involves effective communication. Using checklists and standardized communication tools increases patient safety. An example of standardized communication is the SBAR tool.

The Joint Commission on Accreditation of Healthcare Organizations (JCAHO) has stated the importance of using standardized communication techniques to improve patient safety. There are many communication tools.

- I PASS the BATON

    Intro
    Patient
    Assessment
    Situation
    Safety concerns
    Background
    Actions
    Timing
    Ownership
    Next

- SBAR

  Situation
  Background
  Assessment
  Recommendation

- Ticket to Ride
  Communication tools are commonly used to inform the transporter when the patient moves to another unit. This information can include whether the patient needs oxygen and when the last pain medication was given.

- Time out
  A "time out" is performed before a procedure is started. All team members stop and listen. The patient, procedure, where the procedure is being performed, and other important information are relayed to the team. Every team member is given the opportunity to speak up about any questions or concerns. When the procedure is complete, a debriefing is performed.

Normal vital signs

The frequency of vital signs is specific to the facility. Vital signs are most commonly collected every five to fifteen minutes in phase 1. Vital signs in phase 2 range from every 30 to 60 minutes. At a minimum, vital signs should be taken on arrival and at discharge from phase 2.

- Temperature- Most accurate core measurement is through a pulmonary catheter. The best alternative is the distal esophagus. Other areas to obtain temperature include Nasopharynx, oral, tympanic membrane, temporal artery, axillary, bladder, and rectum. Shivering can increase heat production by 500%.

  Heat loss can occur through radiation- heat moves to a cooler location without the need to touch another object.
  - o Conduction- heat moves through contact with other objects.
  - o Convection- Body heat moves to cooler air.
  - o Evaporation- heat transfers when a liquid is changed into a gas.

  Normothermia - 36-38

  Hypothermia may be a desired condition for some surgeries such as cardiac or brain. This is used to decrease oxygen requirements and metabolic demands. Cardiac events may occur if the temperature is less than 91.4 F (33 C). Unplanned hypothermia may also cause impaired wound healing, increased infection rates, and increased bleeding.

$F= (C \times 9/5) +32$
$C=(F-32) \times 5/9$

- B/P
    - Toddler- B/P 95-105 / 55-66
    - Preschooler- B/P 95-110 / 56-70
    - School-age child- B/P 97-112 / 57-71
    - Adolescent- B/P 112-128 / 66-80

- HR
    - Age 1-2= 80-130
    - Age 3-4= 80-120
    - Age 5-6= 75-115
    - Age 7-9= 70-110

- Respiratory rate

    - Newborn- 36-60
    - Toddler-24-40
    - Preschool 22-34
    - School age 18-30

➢ Capnography: End-tidal Co2- 35-45 measured with capnography

- Can detect early hypoxia to allow correction of hypoventilation, apnea, or airway obstruction.

- It can be used in areas other than the operating room for procedures or peripheral nerve blocks.

- It can increase safety for patients when included with the use of pulse oximetry. Oxygen supplementation may correct for pulse oximetry readings but may mask hypoventilation.

- A sensitive indicator for respiratory acidosis

- Capnography can be measured in intubated and non-intubated patients.

Hemodynamic monitoring- The most common invasive measurements in the PACU are central venous pressure (CVP) and arterial blood pressure. Monitoring is used for critically ill or unstable patients.

- The CVP measures the pressure in the vena cava and estimates preload and right atrial pressure. The CVP can be used to assess vascular volume and cardiac function. Normal values are 3-8 cmH2O. A CVP can be monitored through a central line placed in the subclavian, internal jugular, femoral, or brachial. This is attached to a pressure line that needs to be zeroed. Transducer placement is essential to obtain correct measurements. Venous blood can be drawn from this pressure line. The CVP reading may be elevated if the patient is on positive end-expiratory pressure (PEEP).

- Arterial blood pressure is obtained through an arterial catheter usually placed in the wrist or groin. These are pressure lines that need to be zeroed. Arterial blood gas measurements can be drawn from this pressure line.

- Allen test- Compress both the radial and ulnar arteries on the wrist. The patient makes a fist to squeeze the blood out of the hand. Release the ulnar artery only. The hand should reperfuse within 5 to 10 seconds. If the hand does not reperfuse, the ulnar artery may be damaged. Do not risk compromising the radial artery with an arterial line in this extremity.

- The CVP and arterial blood pressure measurements transducer should be placed at the mid-anterior-posterior diameter of the chest wall at the fourth intercostal space. An easy way to remember this is that it is near the distal edge of the blood pressure cuff on the arm. This area is called the phlebostatic axis, which is at the level of the right atrium. The bed should be elevated 60 degrees or less.

- Patients may be monitored with a Swan-Ganz catheter which is also known as a right heart catheter or a pulmonary artery catheter. Care must be taken to prevent infections. When checking wedge pressures, be sure not to leave the balloon inflated; This can cause necrosis.

  Many variables can be monitored with a Swan-Ganz. Pulmonary artery pressure, central venous pressure, pulmonary artery wedge pressure, and cardiac output are a few.

- Cardiac output (CO)- The amount of blood ejected by the ventricle with each heartbeat. The stroke volume and heart rate affect the CO.

- Preload is the amount of end-diastolic stretch on the cardiac muscle fibers. This is determined by the volume of blood filling the ventricle at the end of diastole.

- Afterload is the resistance or pressure the ventricle must overcome to eject the blood.

- Potential complications with central lines:
  - Infections- Keep the site clean; use a sterile technique to place. Be sure to document the guidewire removal if one is used.
  - Air embolism
  - Thrombus or embolic event
  - Pneumothorax from complications with placement. Obtain a chest X-ray for lines that may cause this.
  - Hematoma
  - The placement of some lines, such as the swan Ganze, may cause cardiac arrhythmias.

- Numbers you may need to know:

  - Right arterial pressure (RAP) - 2-6 mmHg

  - Right ventricular pressure (RVP)- Systolic-15-25 mmHg, diastolic 0-8

  - Mean arterial pressure- Systole plus (2 times diastole) Divided by three. The normal value is 70-105.

  - Pulmonary artery pressure (PAP)- Systolic 15-25 mmHg, Diastolic 8-15.

  - Pulmonary artery wedge pressure (PAWP)- 6-12 mmHg

  - Cardiac output (CO)- 4-8 L/min

- Cardiac index (CI)- 2.5-4 L/min/m2

- Stroke volume index (SVI) 33-47 ml/m2/beat

- Systemic vascular resistance (SVR)- 800-1200 dynes

- CO= Stroke volume multiplied by Heart rate

- **ICP-** Intracranial pressure can also be monitored in the PACU. The surgeon places a sensor into the patient's skull that is attached to a monitor. Usually, there is a device that allows CSF- cerebral spinal fluid- to be drained off if the ICP becomes elevated. The placement of the transducer for ICP measurements is at the tragus of the ear—normal ICP measures 7 – 15 mm Hg.

- To troubleshoot hemodynamic lines, first- always check your patient. If they are stable, then ensure all the connections are intact and nothing leaks. Try flushing the line if appropriate. Make sure the transducer is correctly placed. You may need to zero the transducer.

Dr. Warner Forssmann placed a catheter into his heart to prove it could be done without killing someone. The year was 1929. It just goes to show how bored someone can be without the internet. He only put it into the right atrium though. He won a Nobel prize for doing it and for inventing other heart catheter instruments. Future doctors perfected the technique. In 1970 Dr. Ganz and Dr. Swan developed a balloon-tipped catheter that floats into the pulmonary artery. This is basically what we use today.

Chatterjee, 2009

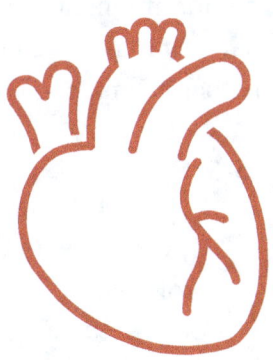

Normal lab values

- BUN-6-20
- Creatinine- Men- 0.6-1.3, Women- 0.5-1.0

- Calcium- Ca- 8.5-10.5
    - Elevated Ca- lethargy, heart block, PVCs, shortened QT interval.
    - Decreased Ca-
        - Positive Trousseau's sign- is a carpal spasm when a blood pressure cuff is inflated on the upper arm to 20 mm Hg for three minutes.
        - Prolonged QT interval
        - Positive Chvostek's sign- a spasm when the face is tapped at the angle of the jaw.

- Hemoglobin males- 14-18
- Hemoglobin females- 12-16
- Hematocrit males- 42-52
- Hematocrit females- 37-47

- K-3.5-5
    - Elevated K can cause flat or absent P waves, wide QRS, peaked T waves, and a prolonged PR interval.
    - Low K can cause flat or inverted T waves, depressed ST, and PVCs.
    - Elevated and decreased K can cause muscle weakness.

- Na- 135-145

- o Elevated Na- Thirst, oliguria
- o Decreased Na- abdominal cramping, nausea, and vomiting.
- o Elevated and decreased Na- Confusion, lethargy, coma, convulsions

- Glucose- 70-110
- WBC-5-10
- Calcium- 8.5-10.2

- PH- 7.38-7.11
- PaCo2- 38-42
- Pao2- 75-100
- HCo3- 23-5

- INR- 1.1 or below
- Platelet -150,000 to 450,000
- PT= Prothrombin time- 9.6-11.8 seconds
- PTT= Partial thromboplastin time- 30-45 seconds

- Magnesium- 1.5-2.2 mEq/L
- Albumin- 3.5-5.5 g/dl

- Troponin- I- 0-0.1 ng/ml- peak 10-24 hours, return to normal in 10 to 14 days after cardiac event. Troponin is found in skeletal and cardiac muscles; Troponin I and T are the cardiac forms. Troponin controls the interaction between myosin and actin.

Normal ABG:

PH: 7.35-7.45
Po2: 80-100 mmHg
Pco2: 35-45 mm Hg
O2 Saturation: 95-97%
Base excess: +2- (-2)
Bicarbonate: 22-26

Urinalysis:

- Blood- RBC- 0-2
- Glucose- 0
- Ketones- 0
- PH-4.6-8.0
- Protein- albumin-0-8mg/dL. The presence may indicate glomerulonephritis.
- Specific gravity- 1.010-1.025. Values decrease with age.
- WBC- 0

Creatinine clearance- Collected for 24 hours and needs to be refrigerated. BUN =10-20, Serum creatinine- 0.5-1.2,

Scoring tools

FLACC pain scale- used to assess pain in children aged 2 months to 7 years. Children are rated from 0 to 2 in five categories for a total score of 0-10.

- Face
- Legs
- Activity
- Cry
- Controllability

CRIES score- Used for neonates to 6 months. A score of 0 is the best, and 10 is the worst.

- Crying,
- Requires O2,
- Increased vital signs from pre-op,
- Expression,
- Sleepless.

Wong-Baker pain scale- Happy face changing to crying face. It can be used for children as young as three years.

Braden scale is a tool to help determine pressure sore risks. This is scored by assessing moisture, activity, mobility, nutrition, friction and shear, and sensory perception.

Aldrete score- this tool is most often used in phase 1 recovery. It was developed in 1970.

- Activity

  2- Able to move all extremities spontaneously or on command

  1- Able to move two extremities spontaneously or on command.

  0- Unable to move any extremities.

- Respiration

  2- Able to deep breathe and cough

  1- Dyspnea, limited breathing

  0- Apneic

- Circulation

  2- B/P within 20 mmHg of pre-op level

  1- B/P within 20-50 mmHg of pre-op level

  0- B/P more than 50 mmHg change from pre-op level

- Consciousness

  2- Fully awake

  1- Awake on calling.

  0- Not responsive

- Skin color

2- Normal

1- Pale, dusky, jaundiced.

0- Cyanotic

Modified Aldrete score replaces skin color with oxygen saturation. This score was developed in 1995, probably due to the fingertip pulse ox monitor becoming widely available at this time. Beginning in 1981, oxygen saturations were monitored in operating rooms and acute respiratory care areas.

- Oxygen saturation

  2- SpO2 greater than 92% on room air

  1- SpO2 greater than 90% with supplemental oxygen

  0- SpO2 less than 90% even with supplemental O2

Glasgow coma scale

- Eye-opening response

  4- Spontaneous

  3- To verbal stimuli

  2- To pain

  1- No response

- Verbal response

  5- Oriented

  4- Confused but able to answer questions

  3- Inappropriate words

  2- Speech incomprehensible

  1- No response

- Motor response

  6- Obeys commands for movement

  5- Responds purposefully to painful stimuli

  4- Withdraws from pain

  3- Flexion in response to painful stimuli

  2- Decerebrate posturing to pain.

  1- No response to pain

Post-anesthesia Discharge Scoring System- PADSS- The total score is 10. A greater than 9 score is typically needed to discharge home.

- Vital signs

  2= Within 20% of the pre-operative value
  1= 20 to 40 % of the pre-operative value
  0= 40% of the pre-operative value

- Ambulation and mental status

  2= Oriented times three and had a steady gait
  1=oriented times three OR has a steady gait
  0= Not oriented, does not have a steady gait

- Pain or nausea/ vomiting

  2=Minimal
  1= Moderate
  0- Severe

- Surgical Bleeding

  2=Minimal
  1= Moderate
  0= Severe

- Intake and output

  2= PO fluids and has voided
  1=Po fluids OR voided
  0= Has not had Po fluids or voided

Modified Postanesthetic Discharge Scoring System (MPADSS)
- Uses the same scoring for vital signs and surgical bleeding but has removed the mental status, intake, and output.

- Ambulation

  2=Steady gait, no dizziness
  1=Ambulates with assistance
  0=Can not ambulate, dizzy

- Nausea

  2=Minimal
  1=Moderate
  0=Severe

- Pain

  2=Minimal
  1=Moderate
  0= Severe

Ramsay sedation scale

Responsiveness	Score
Anxious, agitated, restless	1
Cooperative, oriented	2
Responds to commands only	3
Quickly responds to light tactile stimulation	4
Sluggish response to tactile stimulation	5
No response	6

Infants and children

- Increased surface area decreased mass: Lack of subcutaneous fat can contribute to hypothermia.
- Decreased functional residual capacity.
- Decreased o2 reserves.
- Greater o2 consumption.
- Greater metabolic rate.

Infants are nose breathers and have a large tongue, narrow nasal passages, and a short neck. An infant's head is larger in proportion to the body. Infants may be difficult to intubate due to the trachea having a smaller diameter. The trachea, larynx, and epiglottis are shaped differently than in adults. Uncuffed ET tubes may be used until children are eight to ten years old.

Special considerations for children:
- Facilities may have flavored O2 masks for children.
- Sedation may be given orally. Then, after the patient has relaxed, the IV may be started.
- Parents may be allowed in the OR or PACU areas where family is not normally allowed.
- Children may be fast-tracked to the Phase 2 area.
- Allow children to maintain as much control as possible.

Fetal surgery- Many conditions during pregnancy may now be surgically repaired. This type of surgery may be done for fetal abnormalities, myelomeningocele, twin-to-twin transfusion syndrome, and other conditions. The pre-and post-op nurse should remember they are caring for two patients. Fetal monitoring will be a part of care as well as emotional support for the mother.

Intraosseous infusion access (IO)- IVs can be challenging to place in children, especially in a trauma or code situation. An IO may be placed for the infusion of drugs and fluids. These are most commonly placed with the help of a drill, but some may be placed using just the hand to push the needle into place. Make sure the IO is stabilized and the area is kept clean. The most common location is in the leg, below the knee. This technique is taught in the pediatric life support class. IO placement is becoming more common in the adult population as well.

Developmental stages

There are many theories of development. Below are theories that seem to be the most common in literature and textbooks.

Erickson:

- Birth to 1 year- trust vs. mistrust
- 1 to 3 years- Autonomy vs. shame and doubt. Children want to be more independent and do more for themselves.
- 3 to 6 years- Initiative vs. guilt. Children this age have a big imagination and want to explore the world. Children begin to develop a conscience.
- 6 to 12 years- Industry vs. inferiority. Children enjoy a sense of accomplishment and learn to cooperate with others.
- 12 to 18 years- Identity vs. role confusion. Adolescents become preoccupied with others' perceptions of themselves and experience rapid physical changes.

Piaget:

- Intuitive- Birth to age 2- sensorimotor, governed by sensations. Age 2 to 7- Preoperational- unable to see other perspectives, imagination in play, questioning the world.
- Concrete operational- Aged 7 to 11- able to see points of view other than their own, cannot deal with abstract concepts but is becoming more socialized in thinking.

- Formal operational- Age 11 to 15- more flexible and adaptable, can understand more abstract thinking.

Freud:

- Birth to one year- oral-sensory. The id component of the personality develops during this stage. This drives instincts.
- One to three years- Anal-urethral. The ego component of the personality develops during these ages. This helps block the irrational thinking of the id. This represents the conscious mind.
- Three to six years- Phallic-locomotion. During the preschool years, the superego begins developing. This functions as a moral arbitrator.
- Six to twelve years- Latency
- Twelve to eighteen years- Genital

Maslow's hierarchy of needs focuses on characteristics that contribute to healthy personality development. Lower-level needs such as food and water take precedence. When needs are met, the next level of needs is the priority.

Adolescence

- Fear loss of control, want to be in control.
- They may have poor self-esteem.
- Mood swings
- They May or may not want their parent with them.

The Elderly

- Normal changes include:

  - Increase in body fat.
  - Arteriosclerotic changes, valvular compliance, coronary artery flow, loss of artery elasticity.
  - Delayed drug metabolism. It can cause delayed anesthesia awakening.
  - Decrease in cardiac output.
  - Decreased renal perfusion.
  - Increased risk of clotting disorders such as DVT and stroke.
  - Decreased CNS activity related to reduced blood flow- May cause slower reaction times.
  - Decreased cognitive function- Need more time to learn a concept, may have a shorter attention span.
  - Homeostatic mechanisms may not function as well as when the patient was younger and may have decreased sensitivity to baroreceptors.
  - They may have difficulty regulating body temperatures and be more at risk for hypothermia or heat stroke. GI system changes- decreased salivation and peristalsis.
  - Pancreatic function decreases with a decrease in the ability to metabolize glucose, which can result in glucose intolerance.
  - A decrease in bone marrow production and a decrease in T cell function may have an increase in autoimmune diseases.

When providing discharge instructions, be aware that some elderly patients may not have a support system or the cognitive ability to follow through with care. Transportation may be an issue, as well as financial concerns. These issues may be present in patients of any age, but in the elderly, they may be more of a problem due to the increased risk from coexisting disease processes. Be aware of the laws regarding mandatory reporting of abuse in the elderly in your state. Abuse of older adults can be physical, emotional, or financial.

Pain control in the elderly population can be difficult. Some elderly patients do not accurately report their pain. They do not want to be a bother. Older people may also be at higher risk for kidney and liver damage from aging or other conditions. Pain should be assessed and treated. Pain medications may need to be given more slowly, and the reactions to the medication should be monitored.

Anesthesia Care

ASA- American Society of Anesthesiology uses a classification system to score patients based on physiological conditions that are not related to the surgery. This may also be seen as a PS- physical status classification.

ASA 1 - is a healthy, non-smoking, normal BMI patient.

ASA 2 - is a patient with mild diseases but well controlled/ may be a current smoker. BMI 30 to 40. Other conditions may include mild hypertension, an old MI, or diet-controlled DM

ASA 3 - is a patient with severe systemic diseases such as COPD or poorly controlled diabetes. Other conditions may include morbid obesity or coronary artery disease with angina.

ASA 4 - is a patient with a disease that is a constant threat to life. Examples could include a patient with a recent CVA or MI.

ASA 5 - is a patient not expected to survive without the planned surgery.

ASA 6 - is a brain-dead patient waiting for organ harvest.

Mallampati Airway Classification- The anesthesia provider instructs the patient to open their mouth. The score is given based on what the provider can see.

Anatomic areas are seen by the anesthesia provider- for Mallampati Airway Classification.	Class
Uvula, tonsillar pillars, soft and hard palate	1
Uvula, hard and soft palate	2
The portion of the uvula and hard palate	3
Portion of the hard palate	4

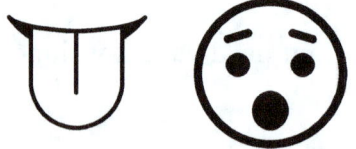

Stages of anesthesia.

Stage 1: Initiation stage. The patient can follow simple commands. Protective reflexes remain intact.

Stage 2: Stage of delirium. The patient loses eyelid reflex, and respiration becomes irregular. During this stage, the neurons that inhibit emotions are not functioning, which causes an excitable state. The patient may experience laryngospasm, emergence delirium, vomiting, or cardiac arrest.

Stage 3: During this stage of anesthesia, the patient experiences loss of spontaneous respiration, blinking, and swallow reflexes.

Stage 4: This is a potentially fatal stage that should not occur. The patient is experiencing an overdose of anesthesia which may lead to circulatory collapse.

A delayed emergence from anesthesia is noted when a patient fails to return to baseline after enough time has passed for the metabolism and elimination of the anesthetic drugs. This condition may be caused by inadequate ventilation and the delivery of oxygen. The patient may not receive adequate stimulation or have an impaired metabolism. Other causes may include cerebral vascular accidents, seizure activity, or prolonged neuromuscular blockade.

Sedation and Nerve Blocks

Sedation

- Minimal sedation, anxiolysis: Patient responds normally. Coordination may be impaired. The patient can maintain the airway.

- Moderate sedation, analgesia: Also known as conscious sedation. The patient has a depressed level of consciousness but can respond to verbal commands or light touch. The patient can maintain their airway.

- Deep sedation, analgesia: Patient responds purposefully to painful stimulation. The patient may not be able to maintain their own airway.

- Anesthesia: General anesthesia- the patient loses consciousness, patients are not arousable, and usually cannot maintain an airway and ventilatory function. Cardiovascular function may be compromised.

o The legal ability for nurses to extubate a patient varies by state. Be aware of specific facility policies if a nurse is responsible for extubating. Extubation criteria include:

- Return of spontaneous respirations 12 to 28 per minute
- Return of protective reflexes
- Absence of respiratory distress
- Ability to lift the head off the pillow for 5 seconds.
- Able to firmly grasp hands.
- Opens eyes on command.

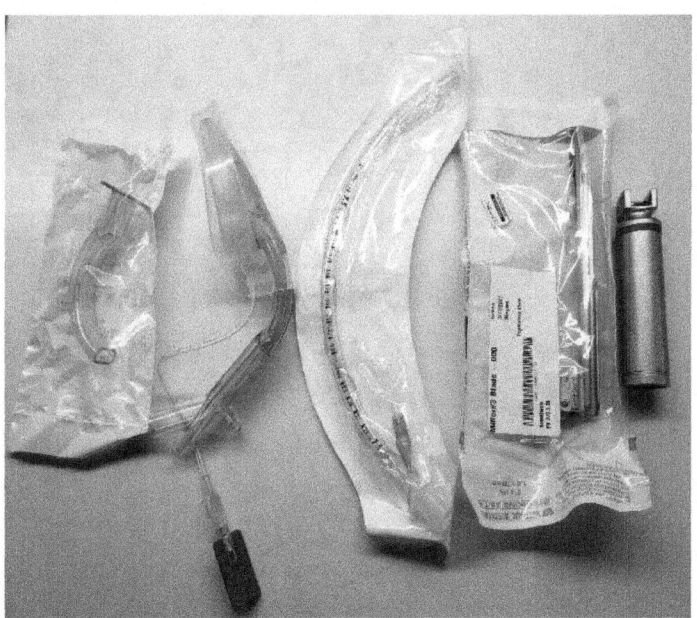

From left to right: OPA- oropharyngeal airway, LMA-Laryngeal mask airway- does not pass the glottis, so it is less invasive than the ET but has a higher risk for aspiration, ET- Endotracheal tube, Laryngoscope, and blade. Miller blades are straight, and Macintosh blades are curved.

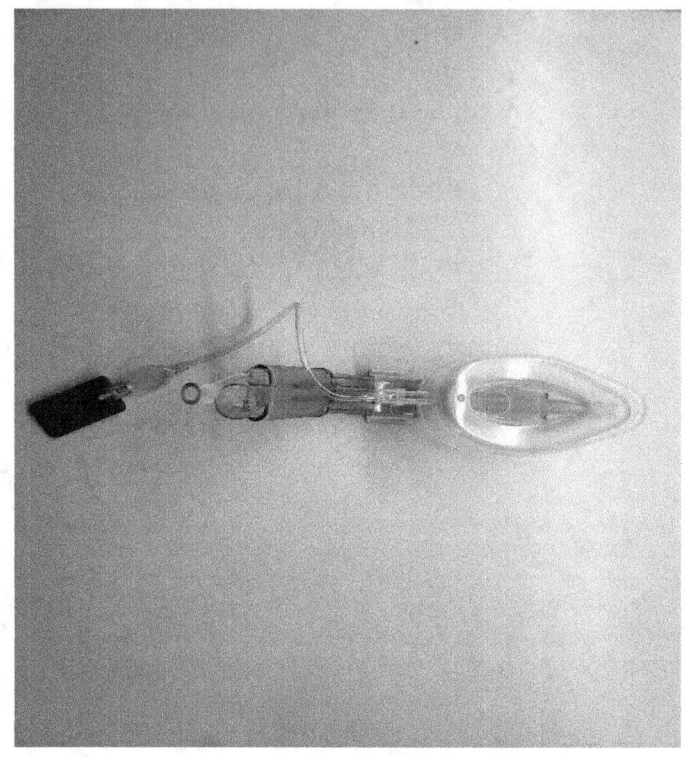

A closer view of a laryngeal mask airway- LMA.

- o Three phases of general anesthesia- Induction, maintenance, and emergence.

- o Oropharyngeal airway- How to measure- Place on the cheek, measure the distance from the mouth's corner to the ear's tragus.

- o Nasopharyngeal airway- How to measure- Nares to the tragus of the ear.

- Regional anesthesia: Loss of sensation to a specific region of the body. Spinal, epidural, and peripheral nerve blocks are examples.

  - Upper extremity: Brachial plexus blocks for shoulder, forearm, or hand surgery. These include inter scalene, supraclavicular, infraclavicular, and axillary.

  - Lower extremity: Femoral, ankle block, and popliteal are examples.

- Local anesthesia: Local infiltration or topical application of the anesthetic agent. An anesthesiologist is usually not needed for these minor procedures.

  - Horner's syndrome- a sign of a medical issue that has caused nerve damage. The nerve from the eye and face to the brain can be damaged and cause drooping eyelids, decreased pupil size, and decreased sweating. A tumor, stroke, spinal cord injury, or as an adverse complication from nerve blocks can cause Horner's syndrome.

  - LAST-Local Anesthetic Systemic Toxicity- Life-threatening adverse reaction to local anesthetics.

- Metallic taste in the mouth
- Periorbital numbness
- Tinnitus
- Dysarthria
- Treat with 20% lipid emulsion.
- ACLS

Nerve blocks

- Retrobulbar- Eye. Used for corneal and lens procedures, commonly performed by the surgeon.

- Intercostal- nerves that supply the ribs and abdominal wall.

- Bier's block-Tourniquet placed on the arm above the surgical site. Medication is placed into an IV placed near the surgical site. There is a possibility of toxicity when the tourniquet is released after the drug is injected.

- Brachial plexus- spinal nerves from C5-T1 vertebrae. Each bundle divides and eventually ends in radial, ulnar, and median nerves. Brachial plexus blocks are used for shoulder, forearm, or hand surgeries.

  o Interscalene- Shoulder surgeries, upper arm
  o Supraclavicular- Elbow and hand
  o Infraclavicular- Elbow, forearm, and hand, but not shoulder
  o Axillary- forearm, wrist, or hand

- Lower extremity nerve blocks are performed for leg, knee, and foot surgeries. Lumbar and sacral nerves divide into sciatic, femoral, popliteal, and tibial nerves.

- o Femoral- For procedures on Anterior thigh and knee arthroscopies and ACL repairs.
  - o Abductor canal- For procedures on the distal thigh, femur, knee, and lower leg.
  - o Ankle- For procedures on foot.

- Abdominal surgeries:

  - o Transverse abdominis plane block (TAP).
  - o Quadratus lumborum (QL)

- Caudal block: Injected into the sacral canal below the dural sac, used for labor pain and surgery below the diaphragm.

Dermatomes are used as a guide to determine anesthetic needs and the extent of a spinal anesthetic. A block higher than T1 may cause cardiopulmonary collapse. A block higher than T3 may cause bradycardia.

- The nipple area corresponds to T4.
- The navel corresponds to T 10
- The groin corresponds to L1.
- The knee corresponds to L4.
- The lateral ankles correspond to S1.

A postprocedural headache may occur in some patients after spinal or epidural anesthesia. The headache may be related to the needle size and the needle's sharpness- blunt needles are less likely to cause headaches, and age- older patients are less likely to experience headaches. A blood patch procedure may be performed to help decrease the headache. This involves drawing a small amount of blood from the patient and injecting it into the patient's back where the leak happened.

> A high spinal may cause cardiac or respiratory complications. Monitor neurologic status, cardiac and respiratory function.

Hypotension may occur after a spinal due to the vasodilation of the vasculature. The patient may experience hypothermia, tachycardia, bradycardia, or hypotension.

A high spinal may cause cardiac or respiratory complications. Monitor neurologic status, cardiac and respiratory function.

To be completed before sedation:

- Pre-sedation evaluation by the anesthesia provider
- Informed consent

- The nurse is relieved of all responsibilities that would prevent that nurse from the ability to constantly monitor the sedated patient.
- Sedation scales:

    o POSS: Pasero Opioid-Induced Sedation Scale- Evaluates sedation and assesses for unwanted sedation. Research has shown this to be the most reliable scoring system based on reliability, validity, and ease of use for nurses.

    o RASS: Richmond Agitation and Sedation Scale- Assessment of sedation in critically ill patients, measures sedation.

    o Aldrete: Determine patients' readiness for discharge from PACU.

    o Ramsey/Modified Ramsey: Assessment of sedation in critically ill patients.

    o Sedation Agitation scale: Assessment of sedation in critically ill patients.

Factors that may contribute to prolonged neuromuscular blockade:

- Acidosis
- Hypokalemia
- Hypercarbia
- Hypothermia
- Metabolic acidosis
- Antibiotics such as tetracycline and aminoglycosides and those that end in "mycin".

Train of Four- TOF- The following numbers are average; you may see different numbers from different sources. The Train of Four is a peripheral nerve stimulator placed on a patient to determine the level of paralysis in an unconscious patient. The device may be placed on the patient's wrist, ankle, or temple. The device is turned on, and the number of times the patient twitches determines the number assigned.

Contractions	Level of paralysis noted as a percent.
0	100%
1	90%
2	80%
3	75%
4	0-75%

If you are asked to help with a procedure, you will need to perform a "Time out." This safety measure is performed before a procedure to ensure it is the correct patient, the correct procedure, the correct site and laterally, and other pertinent information such as the patient's allergy.

Emergency and Difficult Situations

Laryngospasm, airway edema, and other complications of the lungs

The spasm of the laryngeal muscles can cause partial or complete obstruction. Signs and symptoms of this include stridor- a high-pitched crowing noise or an absence of breath sounds. Causes include a substance on the vocal cords, such as blood, mucus, or vomit. Suctioning well before Extubation may prevent this. Conditions that may increase the likelihood of laryngospasm include COPD, smoking, asthma, or trauma. The patient may need medications such as dexamethasone or lidocaine to reduce inflammation. If there is complete obstruction, the patient may need a paralytic such as succinylcholine and to be reintubated.

Bronchospasms- caused by constriction of the bronchial smooth muscles. This may be caused by an allergic reaction, increased secretions, COPD, or asthma. Treatment includes removal of the irritant, increasing O2, albuterol, or medications such as muscle relaxants or hydrocortisone.

Pulmonary edema- This is fluid accumulation in the alveoli. The patient will possibly have frothy pink sputum, dyspnea, wheezing, and hypoxia. Pulmonary edema may be caused by fluid overload, heart disease, prolonged airway obstruction, sepsis, trauma, or transfusion reaction. The patient may need intubation, increased oxygen delivery, diuretics, and muscle relaxants.

Pulmonary Embolus- A blood flow obstruction in pulmonary vessels. It can be caused by a thrombus or fat embolus. This can happen in surgery from fractures and surgery on the long bones. It can occur in pelvic traumas or hypercoagulability conditions. Treatment includes heparin to support breathing. The patient may need intubation. Signs and symptoms:

- A chest X-ray may show a wedge-shaped defect with diaphragmatic elevation.
- Cough
- Dyspnea
- EKG may show T-wave inversion or ST depression.
- Hypotension
- Hypoxia
- Pleuritic chest pain
- Rales
- Restlessness
- Tachycardia
- Tachypnea

Pneumothorax- Can be caused by surgical procedures on the chest, such as the placement of central line catheters. Hypotension and tachycardia can be signs. Treatment is usually the placement of a chest tube.

Emergence Delirium-

The patient wakes up disoriented, demonstrates air hunger, and is "wild." Ensure the patient is not hypoxic. Give oxygen as needed. The patient May need Ativan or a narcotic. Involve parents if the patient is a child or caregiver or family if the patient is an adult. A familiar voice may help calm the patient. Restraints may make the condition worse. Only use restraints when the patient's safety is at risk. Multiple staff members may be needed to prevent the patient from hurting themselves or others.

Malignant Hyperthermia (MH)-

Caused by an autosomal dominant trait causes calcium to be released from muscles. Anesthetic medications can trigger MH, or it can be seen as a reaction to extreme exercise and heat, but this is rare. Family history is taken pre-op to see if there are any unusual surgical deaths or if malignant hyperthermia is known. Most cases occur in healthy patients.

A muscle biopsy is a procedure for diagnosis preoperatively. This is called a caffeine-halothane contracture test. This test is difficult to do as only about 30 labs worldwide conduct the test, and most patients need to go to the site for the test. The test is also known to be expensive.

The total number of patients affected by MH is unknown partially due to the cost and rare cases of testing. A patient may be susceptible but never receives a triggering agent, so the patient may never know. Literature shows a wide range of incidences. Mhaus.org- the Malignant Hyperthermia Association of the United States website states rages from one in 5,000 to one in 100,000. The website states that two to three people die yearly from MH.

MH is a hypermetabolic state of a genetic base that is triggered by medication. MH can occur on induction and up to 24 hours post-medication administration. The signs and symptoms of MH are caused by an excess of calcium ions in the myoplasm. The reuptake of calcium is decreased. This causes the skeletal muscles to contract. Prolonged muscle contraction causes a hypermetabolic state of acid and heat production. The spasm of the masseter muscle is of particular concern causing the mouth to not open for intubation.

As soon as MH is suspected, call for help. Discontinue all triggering agents. Change the anesthesia respiratory circuit and hyperventilate the patient with 100% O2. Know where to find the department's MH cart and bring it to the patient.

- S/S: The first sign is typically an increase in end-tidal CO2.

  - Tachycardia
  - The co2 absorber becomes blue and heated.
  - Tachypnea
  - Increased end-tidal CO2, acidosis
  - Muscle rigidity
  - Mottling of skin
  - Hyperthermia
  - Increased potassium
  - Myoglobinuria
  - Hypertension
  - Hyperkalemia
  - Increased minute ventilation

- Treatment: Know what is in your facility MH cart!

  - Dantrolene - 2.5 mg/kg. Repeat until 10mg/kg. Only dilute with preservative-free sterile water. Dantrolene is a hydantoin skeletal muscle relaxant that also affects the vascular and heart muscle. The mechanism of action is reducing the release of calcium by the sarcoplasmic reticulum without affecting reuptake. Before dantrolene, the mortality rate for malignant hyperthermia was 70%; now, it is around 5%. Most facilities should have 36 vials, diluting each with 60 ML sterile water. There are 3 grams of mannitol in each 20 mg of dantrolene.

o Ryanodex- A new formulation of Dantrolene. Dilute with 5 Ml sterile water. Each facility should have three vials. There are 0.125 grams of mannitol in each vial of 250 mg of Ryanodex.

o Ice packs

o Cold IV solution.

o Sterile water for reconstitution.

o Calcium chloride

o Sodium bicarbonate 8.4%

o Dextrose

o Regular insulin

o Saline- cold. This may be located in the operating room core in a refrigerator.

o Syringes and IV start equipment

o Pressure bag

o Foley with urine meter

o Bucket and plastic bags for ice- Where do you get ice? The PACU ice machine? The coffee bar?

o Drapes to cover the surgical wound.

- Medications that do not cause malignant hyperthermia:

  - Nitrous oxide
  - Opioids
  - Barbiturates
  - Droperidol
  - Pancuronium
  - Propofol
  - Benzodiazepines
  - Ketamine
  - Etomidate
  - Vecuronium

- Medications that may activate malignant hyperthermia:

  - Halothane
  - Enflurane
  - Isoflurane
  - Sevoflurane
  - Desflurane
  - Chloroform- Is used in pesticides, as a solvent, in labs, and in the production of plastics. This is known as toxic and may cause cancer. It was used in the old days as an anesthetic and sedative.
  - Succinylcholine

    Treating symptoms- electrolyte imbalances, cardiac dysrhythmias. The patient may need to be intubated if MH happens after surgical Extubation.

69

After stabilized, send the patient to critical care for at least 24-hour monitoring. Dantrolene can be continued in the post-op areas and is available orally. The patient commonly will have arterial and central lines. Educate patients and families on possible genetic susceptibility.

MHAUS hotline number 1-800-644-9737. Call and place on speaker phone.

Blood transfusion reaction

Stop transfusion. Notify MD. Prepare for possible orders for treatment of symptoms.

- Fever
- Rash
- Dyspnea
- Hypotension
- Bronchospasm
- Anxiety
- Increased interop bleeding
- Weak pulse
- Vasomotor instability
- Decreased urine output.

Types of Transfusion Reactions-

Transfusion reactions can occur up to weeks after transfusion.

- Acute hemolytic reactions- This can happen if there's red blood cell damage before the transfusion due to heat or an imbalance in the cells.
- An anaphylactic reaction is similar to a simple allergic reaction but more severe.
- Delayed hemolytic reactions may happen when an antigen (toxin or foreign substance) gets reintroduced into your blood.
- Febrile non-hemolytic reactions may happen when your donor's white blood cells produce cytokines (substances that work with the immune system).
- Simple allergic reactions. This may happen if your blood is hypersensitive to protein in your donor's blood.
- Transfusion-associated circulatory overload (TACO)- Caused by fluid overload in the body.
- Transfusion-related acute lung injury (TRALI)- Immune system response can lead to pulmonary edema.
- Septic (bacteria contamination) reactions can occur if the donated blood is contaminated with bacteria or bacteria waste products.

Some interesting facts about blood-

Most patients who refuse transfusion, such as Jehovah's Witnesses, will accept their own blood back if it has remained connected to their circulation with a blood salvage machine.

The drug epoetin alfa (recombinant human erythropoietin) stimulates erythropoiesis in the bone marrow.

Hypocalcemia may occur in patients after transfusion due to the ionized calcium binding with the citrate used to preserve stored blood.

Cardiac arrest

Cardiac arrest in the preoperative area, the operating room, and recovery areas can have a variety of causes. Hypovolemia, embolisms, and malignant hyperthermia are possible causes of cardiac dysrhythmias or arrest. Some causes can be corrected preoperatively, such as canceling elective surgeries if the patient has not been optimized. In situations such as trauma, having an adequate blood supply to be transfused may prevent issues.

If your patient experiences cardiac arrest, follow the current guidelines by the American Heart Association. Each facility will have different requirements about what certifications the staff may need to have, such as BLS- basic life support, ACLS- advanced cardiac life support, and PALS-pediatric life support. These certifications last two years and may be provided by the hospital at no cost to the nurse.

A photo of an adult crash/ code cart. There is a monitor/ defibrillator with pads attached. The drawers are labeled for easily finding equipment and medications. Code carts should be centrally located. This cart is supplied with a suction machine.

Operating rooms are also often equipped with a malignant hyperthermia cart which will contain dantrolene, the malignant hyperthermia hotline phone number, and other equipment that may be needed in a MH crisis.

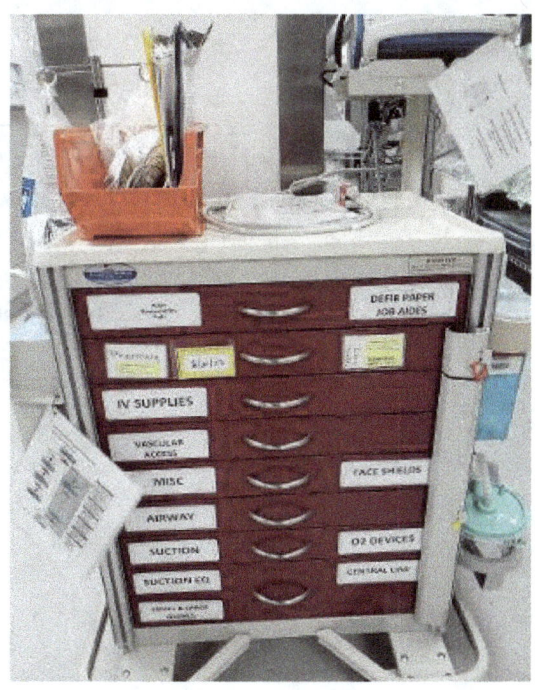

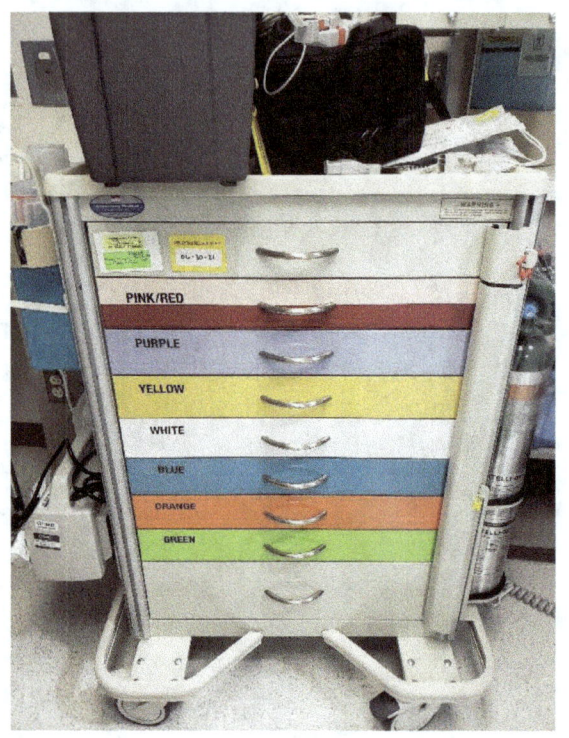

This is an example of a pediatric crash cart. The drawers are color-coded according to the patient's size. These should be located in areas that care for children.

Awareness under anesthesia

Sometimes, patients can remember some or all of the surgical experience. The anesthesia provider should be notified. A Brice questionnaire may be used for the assessment of the recall. Awareness under anesthesia is not common- one to two per thousand patients. Awareness may be pleasant or terrifying and may lead to post-traumatic stress disorder.

Hypothermia

Monitor the patient's temperature on arrival at the PACU and regularly as per your facility guidelines. Give the patient warm blankets or turn on a warming blanket. If possible, infuse warmed IV fluids.

If shivering occurs, the patient may have an increased oxygen demand that may cause ST depression due to increased myocardial oxygen requirement. The patient may demonstrate somnolence due to decreased perfusion to the brain.

Poor wound healing and increased infections are also risks of hypothermia. The patient may also be less comfortable and possibly have more anxiety when cold.

Post-op nausea and vomiting

Factors that may increase the risk:

- Female gender
- History of post-op nausea and vomiting
- History of motion sickness
- Obesity
- Non-smokers
- Use of volatile anesthetics
- Opioids
- Long duration of surgery
- Abdominal procedures
- Ear, nose, and throat surgery if blood enters the stomach.

Post-op nausea and vomiting non-medical treatments can include:

- Aromatherapy with ginger, tarragon, peppermint, or alcohol.
- Supplemental O2.
- Deep breathing
- Cold washcloth to forehead
- Acupuncture

Trauma

Patients may be brought to the operating room from the emergency room after trauma. Trauma may occur from motor vehicle crashes, gunshots, stabbings, falls (Often seen by grandfathers who know better than to get on the ladder), and other mechanisms of injury that necessitate emergency care. The patient may have blunt injuries, stabbing injuries, fractured bones, or other injuries.

The golden hour- Coined by Dr. R. Adams Crowley, MD. This time is considered the optimal window to conduct life and limb-saving procedures.

AMPLE- Allergies, medications, past medical history, last meal, events.

Types of shock:

- Hypovolemic
- Cardiogenic- This may be secondary to blunt trauma.
- Distributive-
  - Neurogenic- May be caused by spinal cord damage or brain trauma. The patient presents with bradycardia and flushed skin.
  - Anaphylactic
  - Septic
- Obstructive- Tension pneumothorax or cardiac tamponade may be the cause.

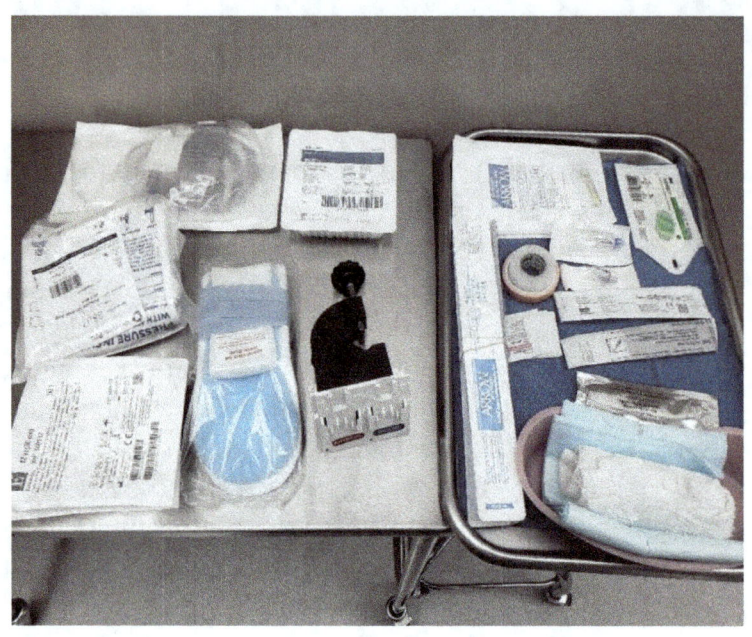

A picture of supplies needed to set up an arterial line. Normal saline is typically used, but your facility may want a heparin solution. Spike the tubing and place the IV fluid in a pressure bag. Inflate the pressure bag. Ensure no bubbles are in the tubing, not even the "Champaign" bubbles. Place the transducer at a level with the patient's phlebostatic axis, which is approximately where the blood pressure cuff is located. Some facilities in the ICU will tape the transducer to the patient's blood pressure cuff, and others will use a construction level to determine placement on an IV pole. Plug in the arterial line to the monitor, turn the stopcock off to the patient (Towards the stiff tubing), open the stopcock to atmospheric pressure, and tap the "Zero" button on the monitor. When the line has been zeroed, turn the stopcock to neutral, place the cap back on, and monitor the patient.

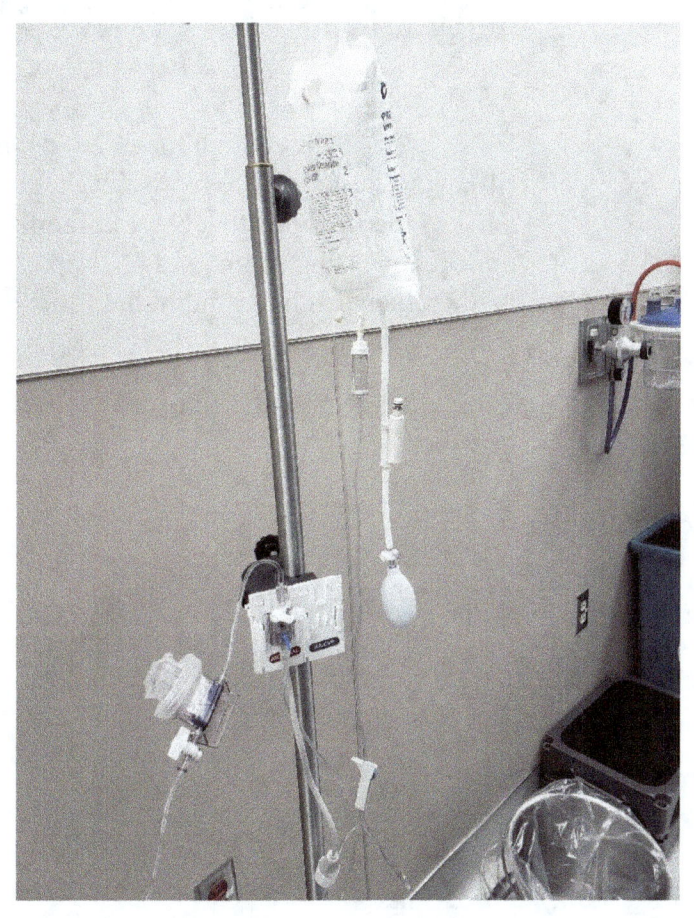

An arterial line is set up and ready to go.

Medications

There are enough medications in the world to fill a very large book. This is not that book. Below is a list of medications that are commonly used in the pre-op, operating room, and post-op areas. More medications can be found in the following surgical category sections.

Remember the rights of medication or treatment:

- Right documentation
- Right dose
- Right drug
- Right patient
- Right reason
- Right route
- Right time

Pain medications

- Acetaminophen- non -opioid; adults should not take more than 4000 mg per 24 hours. It can be toxic to the liver.

- Aspirin- Some patients may take this for pain control. Aspirin inhibits prostaglandin synthesis. Platelets are disabled. It should be stopped before surgery. Platelets can be infused to reverse effects.

- Celecoxib (Celebrex)- Nonsteroidal anti-inflammatory. It can be given pre-op to help prevent post-op pain, commonly used for arthritis.

- Hydromorphone (Dilaudid)- analgesic opioid agonist.

- Fentanyl (Sublimaze)- Analgesic opioid agonists

- Gabapentin (Neurontin)- Analgesic adjunct, anticonvulsant, mood stabilizer.

- Ketorolac (Toradol)- NSAID analgesic.

- Meperidine (Demerol)- Opioid analgesic. It can be used for patients shivering post-op. It can increase intracranial pressure. Do not use in a patient taking MAOI inhibitor. Narcan is the antidote.

- Morphine- Opioid analgesic. Narcan is the antidote.

- Nalbuphine (Nubain)- Opioid analgesic.

- Norco- Acetaminophen plus hydrocodone. Opioid for moderate to moderate-severe pain.

- NSAID- Ibuprofen, Advil, Mortin, Naproxen.

- Oxycodone (Oxycontin) -Opioid analgesic.

- Tramadol- Ultram- Analgesic opioid agonists treat moderate to severe pain.

Anesthesia gasses

- Desflurane- Fluorinated methyl ether, general anesthetic, irritating odor.

- Halothane- General anesthetic. Nonirritating and not bad smelling. It may be used for children.

- Isoflurane (Forane)-General anesthetic. Bad smell, irritating gas.

- Nitrous oxide (N2O)- Anesthetic gas with pain-relieving properties. Short-acting, not a malignant hyperthermia trigger. Smells sweet. Has a weak anesthetic effect. Needs to be mixed with oxygen, not room air, to prevent diffusion hypoxia.

- Sevoflurane- Fluorinated isopropyl ether, general anesthetic. Nonirritating smell.

Neuromuscular blocking agents, paralytics

- Atracurium-Lowers seizure threshold. Store in refrigerator.

- Nimbex (Cisatracurium)- Non-depolarizing neuromuscular blocker. Store in refrigerator. Lowers seizure threshold.

- Pavulon (Pancuronium) can increase heart rate, cardiac output, and mean arterial pressure (MAP).

- Rocuronium- non-depolarizing neuromuscular blocker.

- Anectine (Succinylcholine)- depolarizing agent.

- Norcuron (Vecuronium)- Has minimal hemodynamic effects. It does not need to be refrigerated.

Local Anesthetics

- Bupivacaine (Marcaine, Sensorcaine)- Can be used in epidural or local. Duration of 3 to 10 hours.

- Cocaine- Topical anesthetic, vasoconstrictor. Most commonly used in the nasal mucosa before intubation or surgery. Signs and symptoms of toxicity include hypertension, tachycardia, seizures, and hyperthermia.

- Epinephrine- alpha/beta-agonist, a bronchodilator, vasopressor, Anitiasthmatics. It is added to other local medications to increase the duration of the anesthetic effect.

- Lidocaine (Xylocaine)- Can be given IV for ventricular arrhythmias.

- Procaine (Novocaine)- Used as spinal anesthesia, peripheral nerve block, or local infiltration.

- Ropivacaine (Naropin)- can be topical, local, or epidural. Duration can be as long as 12 hours.

- Tetracaine (pontocaine)- Slow onset, long duration.

Treatment for hypertension

- Amidate (Etomidate)- decreases blood pressure.

- Atenolol (Tenormin)- Beta blocker

- Clonidine- Stimulates alpha 2 receptors in the brain. This medication will decrease cardiac output and peripheral vascular resistance.

- Diltiazem (Cardizem)- Calcium channel blocker

- Doxazosin (Cardura)-peripherally acting antiadrenergic.

- Enalapril- Vasotec- ACE inhibitor

- Hydralazine (Apresoline)- Antihypertensive vasodilator.

- Labetalol (Trandate)- Beta blocker, antianginal.

- Lisinopril- ACE inhibitor

- Metoprolol (Lopressor)- Beta blocker. Decreases B/P and HR.

- Nicardipine- Antianginals, antihypertensive, calcium channel blocker.

- Nifedipine- Calcium channel blocker

- Nitroprusside (Nipride)- Vasodilator. This medication is sensitive to light and may come in a package designed to protect it.

- Verapamil- Calcium channel blocker

Antiemetics and anti-nausea

- Dexamethasone- (Decadron)- Can cause vaginal and anal itching and burning.

- Dimenhydrinare (Dramamine)- May cause dry mouth and urinary retention.

- Droperidol (Inapsine)- Antiemetic with sedative and

- anti-anxiety effects. May cause prolonged QT interval.

- Metoclopramide (Reglan)- Antiemetics. Unlabeled use- treatment of hiccups. Increases GI motility.

- Ondansetron (Zofran)- Antiemetic.

- Prochlorperazine (Compazine, Prochlorazine)- Antiemetic, antipsychotic. May cause dry mouth and urinary retention.

- Promethazine- Synthetic antihistamine used to treat nausea. May also be used for sleep problems or allergy symptoms.

- Scopolamine- Anticholinergic. Patch placed behind the ear to help prevent surgical nausea and vomiting. It can also be given to reduce saliva. Anticholinergic drug. Also known as Devil's breath. That won't be on the test; it's just cool. Warn patients of the possibility of dry mouth. Wash hands after handling- if scopolamine gets in the eye, it may cause dilation of the pupil. Do not give it to patient who have narrow angle glaucoma.

- Ginger and peppermint- Studies have shown they work better than placebo. Some nurses swear by having the patient sniff an alcohol wipe. None of this has ever worked for me, but to each his own.

Reversal agents and antidotes

- Acetylcysteine- Antidote for acetaminophen.

- Flumazenil (Romazicon)- Reverses effects of benzodiazepines.

- Narcan- Opioid antagonist.

- Neostigmine- Reversal for non-depolarizing muscle relaxant.

- Sugammadex- Neuromuscular reversal drug. Reverses the non-depolarizing muscle relaxants such as rocuronium and vecuronium. Female patients of childbearing age should be cautioned to use a backup birth control method if on birth control pills. Expensive.

- Protamine- reverse effects of heparin. Derived from fish. It can cause hypotension and pulmonary hypertension.

- Sodium bicarbonate- Management of metabolic acidosis. It may be given in emergency situations. It can be used in an overdose of aspirin and phenobarbital to promote excretion.

- Vitamin K- Phytonadione (Mephyton, Vitamin K)- reverse effects of Coumadin-Warfarin.

Anticoagulants

- Apixaban (Eliquis)- Anticoagulant. The antidote is andexanet alfa. Oral-activated charcoal can decrease absorption.

- Coumadin- warfarin- Often discontinued 48 hours before surgery.

- Dabigatran (Pradaxa)- Thrombin inhibitor.

- Dalteparin (Fragmin)- Anticoagulant. Low molecular weight heparin.

- Enoxaparin (Lovenox)- Anticoagulant. Low molecular weight heparin.

- Eptifibatide (Integrilin)- Antiplatelet agent.

- Heparin- Anticoagulant, antithrombotic. Protamine is an antidote.

- Clopidogrel (Plavix)- Antiplatelet agent. often used for patients with coronary stents

- Rivaroxaban (Xarelto)- Anticoagulant, antithrombotic.

Antibiotics/anti-infective/ antifungal

- Amoxicillin
- Amphotericin B- Antifungal
- Cefazolin- (Ancef)- Cephalosporin first generation.
- Ceftriaxone –(Rocephin)- Cephalosporin third generation
- Ciprofloxacin
- Clindamycin
- Erythromycin
- Gentamycin
- Imipenem- Anti-ineffective.

- Metronidazole (Flagyl)- Anti-infectives, antiprotozoals.
- Piperacillin (Zosyn)- Extended-spectrum penicillin.
- Tetracyclines
- Vancomycin

Diuretics- Usually held on the day of surgery unless the physician wants to continue, usually for CHF or renal failure.

- Bumetanide (Bumex)- Loop diuretic
- Ethacrynic acid (Edecrin)- Loop diuretic
- Furosemide (Lasix)- Loop diuretic
- Mannitol (Osmitrol)- Osmotic diuretic
- Spironolactone (Aldactone)- Potassium sparing
- Torsemide (Demadex)- Loop diuretic

Herbs- Herbs are not regulated: with the exception of the removal of herbs that are proven to be unsafe. There is no proof of efficacy for herbs. Reporting adverse effects is unreliable. Common herbs that may be taken by patients are listed below, with known possible adverse reactions.

- St. John's wart- may prolong anesthesia.

- Echinacea- Taken for anti-inflammatory and immunity. It may inhibit hepatic enzymes and affect anesthetic agents.

- Ephedra- Also known as Ma Huang, taken for weight loss and to increase energy. It may cause hypertension or arrhythmias. It should not be given with halothane.

- Fish oil- Taken for anti-inflammatory effects and to reduce cholesterol. It may have an anticoagulant effect and inhibit platelet aggression.
- Garlic, ginkgo, and ginger- Taken to prevent cancer and lower the risk of atherosclerosis. Also, for antispasmodic and anti-inflammatory. It may cause post-op bleeding.

- Ginseng- Can increase blood pressure and heart rate.

- Valerian- Taken for insomnia. It can increase the effects of anesthesia and prolong patient recovery and "Wake up" from surgery.

Obstetrical

- Magnesium- Can be given via IV for hypertension, common in post-delivery in women.

- Mifepristone (Mifeprex)- Abortifacients. Termination of pregnancy. It can be used for cervical ripening. It may cause uterine rupture.

- Misoprostol (Cytotec)- Can be used to prevent gastric ulcers or terminate pregnancy.

- Oxytocin (Pitocin)- Oxytocic. Help the uterus contract after delivery or induction of labor.

- RhoGAM- Derived from human plasma. It helps prevent Rh immunization, also called Rh incompatibility. Given to people who are Rh negative but receive blood products that are Rh positive or to women who are Rh neg and may be pregnant with a fetus who is Rh positive.

Emergency medications

- Adenosine- Antiarrhythmic. Given for paroxysmal supraventricular tachycardia.

- Amiodarone- Antiarrhythmic.

- Atropine- Anticholinergic. Given for treatment of brady arrhythmias.

- Dantrolene (Ryanodex)- Skeletal muscle relaxant. Treatment for malignant hyperthermia

- Esmolol (Brevibloc)- Antiarrhythmic.

Common medications that are given by the anesthesia provider

- Etomidate- Used as an anesthetic induction agent.

- Glycopyrrolate- Reduces secretions. Anticholinergic. Used to control heart rate. Non-surgical use includes control of peptic ulcers. Anticholinergic drugs can cause tachycardia and dry mouth.

- Ketalar (Ketamine)- Dissociative anesthetic. It can increase heart rate and blood pressure. It can cause hallucinations. Used as an anesthetic induction agent.

- Midazolam (Versed)- Benzodiazepine, anticonvulsant, sedative-hypnotic.

- Phenylephrine (Neo-Synephrine)- Alpha-adrenergic. Causes vasoconstriction, decreased heart rate, and increased blood pressure.

- Propofol (Diprivan)- General anesthetic. Short-acting causes loss of consciousness and lack of memory. It can be given In an IV drip for a patient on ventilators in the ICU.

- Norepinephrine (Levophed)- Vasopressor. Treatment of severe hypotension.

Miscellaneous

- Albuterol- Bronchodilator.

- Dobutamine- Inotropic, adrenergic- For management of heart failure. Increases cardiac output without increasing heart rate.

- Dopamine- Inotropic, vasopressor, adrenergic. Increases renal perfusion, B/P, and cardiac output. Extravasation can cause sloughing of tissue.

- Epoetin- Stimulates the production of red blood cells.

- Haloperidol (Haldol)- Antipsychotic. It may be given post-op for nausea and vomiting.

- Hetastarch (Hespan)- Plasma expander.

- Lorazepam (Ativan)- Benzodiazepine. Decreases anxiety.

- Monoamine oxidase inhibitor (MAOI)- Antidepressants. It may be held for surgery due to the possible reaction with anesthetic drugs to cause the release of epinephrine and dopamine.

- Milrinone- Inotropic. Short-term treatment of heart failure.

- Mitomycin- Treatment for cancer. Often used for bladder cancer. The surgeon may place in the patient's bladder via a foley to be left for a specific amount of time. The recovery room nurse may then empty the bladder and remove the foley.

- Nitroglycerine- Used to prevent chest pain and can lower blood pressure.

- Oxybutynin (Ditropan)- For overactive bladder. Urinary tract antispasmodic.

- Precedex (Dexmedetomidine)- sedative, hypnotic. Relax smooth muscle.

- Rifampin- Can be given to TB patients. It can turn urine, tears, and other secretions orange.

- SSRI- Selective serotonin reuptake inhibitors. These medications may slow the hepatic clearance of anesthetic drugs.

- Sucralfate (Carafate)- Antiulcer agent, GI protectant.

- Tranexamic acid- Helps decrease blood loss. Inhibits fibrinolysis.

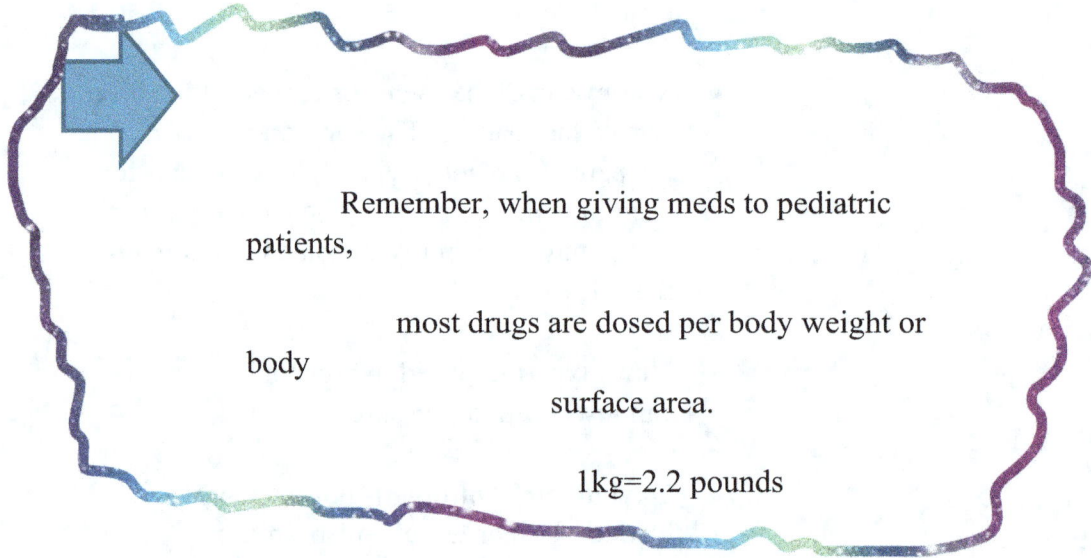

Remember, when giving meds to pediatric patients,

most drugs are dosed per body weight or body

surface area.

1kg=2.2 pounds

Medications commonly allowed to be taken on the day of surgery:

- Antiarrhythmic
- Calcium channel blockers
- Clonidine

- Heart failure medications
- Nitrates
- Pulmonary hypertension medications
- Statins

Medications commonly held for surgery:

- Psychotropic agents- This class of medications can react with anesthesia and cause adverse effects. Medications may need to be tapered off before surgery.

- Ace inhibitors- Commonly held 24 hours before surgery.

Alternative therapies:

- Acupuncture- Based on Chinese medical theory, involves needles placed in specific body areas.
- Ayurvedic- Traditional Hindu medicine. Restores balance using herbs, massage, diet, exercise, and other techniques.
- Balneotherapy- Baths
- Qigong- Traditional Chinese medicine uses meditation, movement, and breathing techniques.
- Reiki- Traditional Japanese involves universal life energy.

Conditions that may affect surgery

Bariatric patients- Nurses need to know the weight limits of beds and other equipment, such as lifts and slings. Special beds may need to be ordered. Obese patients are at risk for hypertension, type 2 diabetes, dyslipidemia, obstructive sleep apnea, and cardiac and peripheral vascular disease.

There are many bariatric surgeries that may be provided depending on your facility and the surgeon's preference. Banding, stimulator implantation, bypass, and diversion methods may be used. The procedure may be performed laparoscopically, open, or robotically. Follow the surgeon's orders on a diet following the surgery. The patient will also typically need to make lifestyle changes. Nutrition deficiencies may occur after surgery. Educate the patient on any supplements that may be needed.

Cystic Fibrosis- Inherited autosomal recessive disorder. These patients experience chronic airway obstruction and exocrine pancreatic insufficiency. The sweat test is used to diagnose cystic fibrosis. These patients should be monitored for airway clearance and infection control.

Myasthenia gravis-An autoimmune disease progressively causing voluntary muscle weakness. Patients may have trouble swallowing, bowel and bladder complications, and difficulty with speech. Watch for aspiration. Classified by type- type 1-4. These patients will likely require prolonged ventilatory support after surgery. May use epidural analgesia to help prevent respiratory depression.

Muscular dystrophy- Progressive degeneration of muscle. May experience respiratory depression after surgery. Encourage coughing and deep breathing. Succinylcholine is contraindicated due to hyperkalemia.

Parkinson's- Continue levodopa. Therapeutic effects may be lost if the drug is stopped for even 6 to 12 hours. Levodopa may cause orthostatic hypotension, dysrhythmias, or hypertension. Do not give these patients phenothiazine (Compazine), which may cause extrapyramidal effects. Ketamine may cause an exaggerated sympathetic response. Patients with Parkinson's may not experience dementia but may have depression symptoms. Check with the patient before surgery to determine if the patient is on MAOI drugs.

Multiple sclerosis- Autoimmune demyelinating disease that affects the spinal cord and brain. Hyperthermia, hypothermia, trauma, surgery fatigue, and emotional stress may cause an exacerbation of symptoms. Succinylcholine may cause hyperkalemia.

Sickle cell anemia- Factors that can cause sickling include hypoxia, acidosis, hypothermia, dehydration, pain, and infection.

Spinal cord injury- The location of the injury can determine the extent of the disability. These patients are possibly at a higher risk for skin breakdown and infection if an indwelling urinary catheter is required. DVT may be an increased risk if the patient has mobility issues. Orthostatic hypotension may be an additional complication for injuries above T7.

Injuries above T6 can increase the risk for autonomic dysreflexia, which is a potentially life-threatening condition with the abnormal overreaction of the autonomic nervous system. Signs and symptoms can include a sudden increase in blood pressure, bradycardia, blurred vision, flushing, and sweating. Bladder distention is the most common cause. Other causes can be pain, fractures, sexual intercourse, and head trauma.

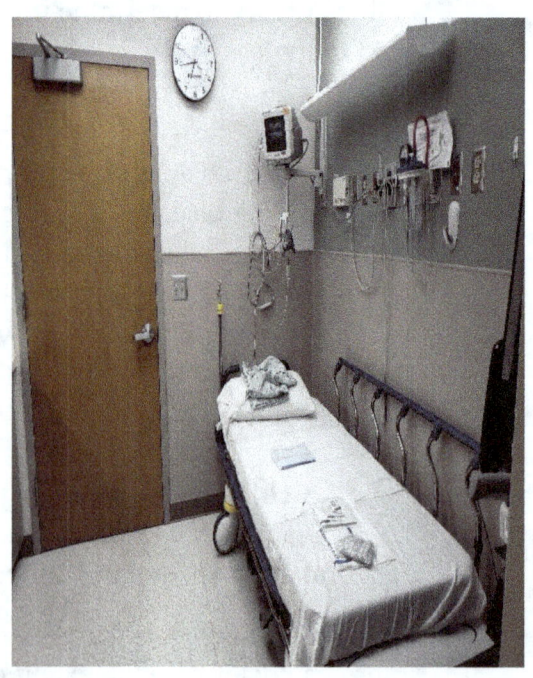

Wound Healing

Anatomy of the skin-

- Epidermis- Outer layer of the skin. Blood is supplied by the dermis. Has sweat glands, sebaceous glands, and hair follicles.
  Five layers of keratinocytes-
  - Stratum corneum- Protects the body from microorganisms and chemical irritants.
  - Stratum lucidum
  - Stratum granulosum
  - Stratum spinosum
  - Stratum Basale- necessary for spontaneous healing.

- Dermis- Layer of skin under the epidermis. Supports the epidermis and provides sensation and temperature control. Two layers of the dermis- Papillary and hypodermis.

Process of wound healing-

- Inflammation- Hemostasis from the vascular response. Thromboplastin is released to activate clotting. Cellular response to help with infection control.

- Proliferation- This begins several days after injury and lasts for several weeks.

- Neovascularization- Formation of new blood vessels
- Epithelialization- Epithelial cells to the wound.
- Collagen formation- Add strength to the healing wound.
- Granulation tissue formation- Connective tissue fills in the wound.

- Remodeling- Scar forms. This stage lasts 1-2 years.

Factors that may affect wound healing include infection, comorbidities, the presence of foreign bodies, and wound size. Children generally heal faster than adults. Older adults may have comorbidities and decreased circulation, which may decrease wound healing. Malnutrition may slow wound healing.

General Surgery

Pre-operative teaching may include:

- Important paperwork to bring includes insurance cards, medication lists, advance directives, and any paperwork from the doctor's office.
- Driving is not permitted postoperatively. The patient will need to make sure transportation has been arranged.
- The patient must be NPO, including gun, candy, and chewing tobacco. These products can increase secretions.
- Wear comfortable clothing that can go over any possible casts or incisions.
- If indicated, teach how to use the CHG bath.
- Make-up and painted fingernails may interfere with some medical devices, such as the O2 saturation monitor or products used to keep the eyes shut during surgery.
- Reminders to fill pain medicine prescriptions if given preoperatively.
- Bring a book or tablet for entertainment in case the case is delayed.
- If hair removal is necessary for surgery, clip the hair, and don't shave. Discourage the patient from shaving at home. Shaving can cause cuts and nicks. Clip the patient as close to the surgical time as possible. Clipping should not be performed in the operating room if possible due to the possibility of

hair contaminating the surgical field. Clip as little hair as necessary. Try to avoid clipping the eyebrows as they do not always grow back well.

Post-operative care for patients depends on the patient and the surgery performed. Post-operative instructions need to be individualized for each patient. All surgeries have risks of infection. Patients are often told they may not bathe or get the surgical site wet for a time after surgery to help prevent infection. Some patients may need to be reminded not to take off the dressing until told to by the surgeon or to wait until the post-op visit. Some patients may also want to rub their family's secret ointment on the wound to help it heal faster. If signs and symptoms of infection occur, the patient needs to understand how and who to notify.

Depending on the surgery and the anesthetic, the patient may have difficulty voiding after surgery. Some surgeries involving the urethra or surgeries with a spinal anesthetic may need to void before discharge. These patients may experience difficulty voiding even after going home and need to understand who to call for help or to go to the emergency department.

Abdominal surgery or drugs may prevent the patient from deep breathing. The patient should be encouraged to cough and deep breathe to prevent atelectasis and other respiratory problems.

Postoperatively, the focus for all types of surgery is the prevention of infection. The patient may need to be told not to put ointments or "grandma's special medicine" on the wound. Tub baths, swimming, and hot tubs are contraindicated for most surgeries. Showering may be allowed depending on the procedure. Give specific information on what to look for and report signs of infection such as an increased temperature, pus, and strange colors.

Some patients may be embarrassed to ask about resuming sexual activity after surgery. Include the information in the postop instructions so they don't have to ask.

Some facilities call the patient at home a day or two after surgery to check on them and ensure the discharge instructions are clear. Some patients are anxious or in pain and will not remember instructions. It is a good idea to teach the patient's family and the patient if the patient allows it.

Laparoscopic surgeries can decrease the time the patient has to stay in the hospital. This surgery involves making several small cuts in the abdomen, where cameras and other instruments can enter. This may also decrease the risk of infection, decrease pain, and allow the patient to get out of bed sooner than traditional open procedures.

Robotic surgeries are becoming more and more popular. The benefit of doing surgery laparoscopically have benefits over open surgery, and robotic surgeries have some benefits over laparoscopic surgeries. The patient may have even shorter recovery times. Disadvantages of robotic and laparoscopic surgeries include a possibly longer surgical time, and they are usually more expensive.

Endoscopic procedures in the abdomen may use a veress needle to introduce a gas, most commonly CO_2, to inflate the abdomen so the surgeon has easier visualization. The insertion of a camera allows for the internal structures to be seen on a video monitor. Pictures can be taken this way to record the procedure. Complications may include

CO_2 being absorbed into the patient's circulation, which may cause hypercarbia and dysrhythmias. The pneumoperitoneum may also cause an increase in abdominal pressure, which may cause respiratory complications such as atelectasis and aspiration. An embolus of CO_2 may cause cardiac complications.

Patients may complain of shoulder pain after laparoscopic procedures. This is caused by the irritation of the diaphragm during surgery. The patient can't "fart it out." Instruct the patient to take pain medication as ordered and avoid carbonated beverages. The feeling will improve with time.

Patients may need to be placed in the Trendelenburg position during surgery. This position can increase the risk of aortic compression, increase mean arterial pressure, pulmonary artery pressure, and a drop in cardiac output.

Lymph nodes- A system closely related to the circulatory system that functions as a transport system moving the lymph from interstitial spaces to the venous bloodstream. This system helps prevent disease and trap foreign matter. It can become enlarged, infected, or involved with metastatic cancer.

Many types of cutting and cauterizing tools are used. A laser is an acronym for light amplification by stimulated emission of radiation. Lasers can cut, coagulate and vaporize tissue. Types of lasers include argon, CO_2, diode and krypton, and others. Laser safety needs to be recognized as lasers can bounce off metal objects and into staff or patients' eyes. Special goggles must be worn by staff that are effective against the type of laser used. A patient's eyes can be protected by special covers such as moist gauze or eyewear. Windows in the operating room should be covered as well to protect those outside the room.

A Bovie is a type of electrosurgical unit that is used to cut and coagulate tissues. This is a monopolar device that requires a grounding pad to be placed on the patient. A bipolar unit also can cut and coagulate but does not need a grounding pad, as the electricity delivered is returned to the same unit.

Deep vein thrombosis (DVT) is a risk for most surgeries. The patient may be at risk due to the length of surgery or being immobile postop. Lower extremity pain, edema, or erythema may indicate DVT. The patient may be given SCD- sequential compression devices for the legs to help blood flow or be placed on an oral or subcutaneous injection of an anticoagulant.

- Virchow's triad- Intervascular vessel wall damage, venous stasis, and a hypercoagulable state

Chest tubes

A patient may present to the PACU with a chest tube. General postoperative care includes ensuring all connections are secure, monitoring for air leaks, keeping the collection device below the chest level, and not clamping unless instructed by the surgeon. Auscultate lung sounds and monitor for atelectasis, pneumothorax, pulmonary edema, and respiratory distress. Palpate around the chest tube insertion site for crepitus, also known as subcutaneous emphysema.

Breast surgery

Breast surgery may be psychologically devastating for a patient. The fear of malignancy, death, changes in body image, and potential negative reactions from family and friends may affect the patient. A patient may also be admitted for reconstructive surgery such as implants, breast reduction, or surgery for cosmetic reasons after surgery for cancer.

Post-op care involves emotional support as needed. Depending on the amount of tissue taken, the patient may have a drain in place and may need post-operative teaching to care for the drain at home. A breast binder may be in place, or the patient may be told to wear a supportive bra without wires.

Papilloma- Grows in a duct. It may cause bloody nipple discharge.

Tumors:

- Benign- may include pain, change in breast size, palpable mass, freely moveable.
- Malignant- May not be painful, fixed mass.

Procedures on the breast:

- Biopsy:
    - Needle
    - Incisional
    - Excisional- Entire mass is removed. It may require needle localization to locate mass accurately.

- o Sentinel node- This can help determine the need for further treatment—node identified by injecting radioisotope.

- Incision and drainage- Patients are usually lactating.

- Partial mastectomy- May be called lumpectomy, segmental, or quadrant resection.

- Subcutaneous mastectomy- Removal of all breast tissue leaving skin and nipple intact.

- Simple mastectomy

- Radical mastectomy- removes all breast tissue, lymph nodes, and muscle of the chest. Rarely done now, but at one time was the standard of care.

- Tissue expanders- Used to stretch normal tissue to provide an area to place implants.

- A flap such as the myocutaneous flap may be used for breast reconstruction. These flaps contain skin, fat, and muscle. The latissimus dorsi and the TRAM flap use this technique.

- Nipple reconstruction may be done at the time of reconstruction, or the surgeon may wish to wait for healing to ensure the new nipple will be placed in the correct anatomical position. Donor sites may be the other nipple, the groin, the buttock, or the auricle. A tattoo may be placed to attempt to make the new nipple appear natural.

Burns

There are multiple tools available to determine the severity of burns.

o   Rule of 9s- The body is divided into equal multiples of 9.
o   Berklow's method and Lund and Browder's chart are used for children.
o   One percent method- Used for a quick assessment.

Burns that involve the face, genitals, electrical burns, or burns accompanied by inhalation injuries may complicate care.

The depth of the injury is assessed.

o   Superficial affects the epidermis. These burns are painful but heal in a few days usually. A sunburn is a superficial burn.

o   Partial thickness- Affects the epidermis and part of the dermis. The skin appears red, moist, blistered, and may have white or yellow areas. Longer healing time may be a month or more.

o   Full thickness- May extend down to the subcutaneous tissue or bone. Has the appearance of leathery black or tan. May not have pain. May need skin grafting.

The patient may demonstrate shock due to the massive fluid loss and shifts causing vasodilation. Sodium and protein are lost from the intravascular space into the interstitium. The patient may easily become hypothermic due to the injured skin's inability to regulate temperature.

Hypothermia and hypovolemia may cause cardiac issues. Catecholamine release may also cause vasoconstriction and increase systemic vascular resistance.

Airway complications may occur if the patient has inhalation injuries or if the chest is burnt, causing decreased airway compliance or shallow breathing due to pain.

Skin grafts may be needed. Grafts may be taken from the patient, cadavers, or a synthetic graft may be used. Skin graft donor sites may be more painful than the burn site.

An escharotomy may be performed when the burn is a circumferential full-thickness burn. The burn may act as a tourniquet and may constrict blood flow. The nerve endings may be dead, so anesthesia may not be necessary.

Skin grafts-

Split thickness- Affects the epidermis and part of the dermis. This type of graft heals faster than a full thickness but may experience contracture.

Full thickness- Contains both dermis and epidermis. Longer healing time than a split thickness but less likely to experience contracture. A full-thickness graft is better to withstand trauma, looks more like real skin, and is better for places of flexion.

Composite graft- Skin and underlying tissues that are separate from the blood supply of the donor site. These types of grafts may be used in hair transplants.

Flap- All or part of the blood supply is intact. May be placed in areas with poor blood supply with full thickness loss. It may be used to cover exposed bone or tendons.

Medications for burns-

Silver sulfadiazine- For wound healing and infection prevention. Applied as a topical cream. It may be painful to apply.

Silver Nitrate- Wound healing and infection prevention. Applied as a topical cream. It may be painful to apply. Does not penetrate eschar well.

GI procedures-

GI procedures may be done in a special unit that only provides GI care. These units may be called same-day, ambulatory care, or simply GI unit. Even if your facility has a special unit for these procedures, GI scopes may sometimes need to be brought into the operating room to assist with surgeries on the GI tract. See the GI section of this book for more information.

Anoscope- A speculum is used to examine the anus.

Colonoscopy- Visualization of the GI tract from the rectum to the ileocecal valve.

Endoscopic retrograde cholangiopancreatography (ERCP)- For visualization of the pancreatic ducts, hepatic ducts, and common bile ducts.

Esophagogastroduodenoscopy (EGD)- For visualization of the esophagus, stomach, and proximal duodenum.

Liver biopsy- Monitor patient post-op for bleeding, fluid leaking, and subcutaneous emphysema.

Paracentesis- To remove fluid to reduce pressure or obtain an abdominal fluid biopsy. This is done for patients with ascites.

Percutaneous endoscopic gastrostomy (PEG)- A feeding tube placed in the stomach through the abdominal wall. Feeding tubes may also be placed in the jejunum- PEJ.

Replantation of an amputated body part

Ideally the amputated body part will be reattached withing 4 to 6 hours. Place the body part in a saline soaked gauze, in an occlusive bag, then place in iced saline.

Toes may be transplanted to the hand in cases of hand damage.

Other General Procedures

Abdominoplasty- Cosmetic procedure used for patients who have lost a large amount of weight and who are having mobility issues due to excessive skin. Compression garments may need to be worn post-op. Body contouring procedures may be performed on other body parts for similar reasons. The patient may have drains and may need teaching to care for drains at home.

Some surgeons consider circumferential abdominoplasty to have a high complication risk, including delayed wound healing and infection.

Cleft lip/ palate- Rule of 10s- at least 10 weeks old, at least 10 pounds, hemoglobin 10 g/dL. Watch for signs of intracranial pressure; elevate the head of the bed and have suctioning equipment available.

Hernia- A defect in the abdominal wall can allow a sac lined by the peritoneum to protrude. Hernias can occur in naturally weak areas such as the inguinal canals, the femoral ring, or the umbilicus. A hernia may also occur where the patient has had an incision in the past.

Rhytidectomy- Known as a face lift. The skin of the face becomes loose in the jowl. Jowl is a weird word. The patient requires their ears to be protected during surgery to prevent fluids from entering the ear canal and protect the eyes from inadvertent damage from instruments.

Cardiac

Cardiac surgery may be performed in a hybrid operating room. These operating rooms combine surgery with interventional radiology. Often, cardiac surgery is performed in its own area of the hospital by dedicated staff with specially trained PACU nurses. I have also seen cardiac surgery patients taken directly to the cardiac intensive care unit to be recovered by intensive care nurses. Cardiac care has changed significantly since I have been a nurse. Surgeries that in the past would have been considered major surgery with multiple days of hospital stay can now be done with the patient going home the same day. This section will briefly touch on some aspects of cardiac care.

Anatomy

The cardiac wall has three layers-

- o Epicardium- Outer lining
- o Myocardium- Muscular layer
- o Endocardium- Inner layer

New York Heart Association's Functional Classification System:

- Class 1- A patient with cardiac disease does not experience symptoms with ordinary physical activity.
- Class 2- Patients with cardiac disease experience symptoms with ordinary activity.
- Class 3- Patients with cardiac disease are comfortable at rest but experience symptoms with minor activity.
- Class 4- Patients are unable to engage in any activity without symptoms.

Medications used for cardiac surgery.

- Heparin- anticoagulant
- Protamine- reverses heparin
- Papaverine- antispasmodic
- Hemostatic agents such as gelatin, collagen, or cellulose
- Sealant- such as coseal, becomes a gel when applied topically.

Anesthetics may affect heart rhythms. Desflurane, isoflurane, and sevoflurane may cause junctional rhythms and/or increase ventricular automaticity. These may also slow the rate of SA node discharge and prolong the conduction times between the bundle of His-Purkinje and ventricular conduction times.

Hypothermia during cardiac surgery- A body temperature of 82.4 F (28C) can reduce oxygen consumption by 50%.

Intra-aortic balloon pump- a device placed in the femoral artery which uses counter pulsation to help increase coronary artery blood flow.

Ventricular assist device- VAD- may be internal or external. Decrease the workload of the heart by diverting the blood flow from the ventricle or ventricles to an artificial pump that maintains systemic perfusion.

Ankle-brachial index- A measurement for arterial perfusion in an extremity. This is an easy bedside assessment. It may be requested by the vascular surgeon pre- and post-operatively.

1. Obtain B/P in both arms. Use the higher reading of the two.
2. Obtain ankle B/P
3. Divide the systolic ankle pressure by the systolic brachial pressure.

Normal= greater than 0.95

Early asymptomatic disease- less than 0.90

Advanced- less than 0.60

Sign of calcified artery- greater than 1.3

Glossary-

Allograft- Tissue from another human, usually a cadaver.

Afterload- The resistance the heart must overcome to pump.

Arteriosclerosis- Thickening and loss of elasticity in arterial walls.

Cardiac index- Cardiac output with considerations for body size.

Cardiac output- The amount of blood ejected by the left ventricle per minute. Measured in liters. Normal value 3 to 6 liters.

Cardioplegia- Paralysis of the heart. Caused by medications, potassium is the most common. This is done to allow surgeons to operate on the heart.

Ejection fraction- An indicator of ventricular function. It is a percentage of end-diastolic volume ejected into the systemic circulation. Normal value- 60% to 70%.

Preload- The pressure and volume of blood in the ventricle at the end of diastole. Central venous pressure is a measure of the right side of the heart, pulmonary artery wedge pressure is a measure of the left side of the heart.

Procedures

Cardiac catheterization- Procedure for determining location of ischemic disease and to diagnose valvular disease. A catheter is placed through the aortic valve into the left side of the heart by a percutaneous puncture. The brachial or femoral artery may be used. Contrast may be used, monitor for renal function.

Coronary artery bypass graft (CABG)- A graft is connected to the artery distal to a narrow section of an artery. This procedure will increase blood flow to the ischemic areas.

Percutaneous coronary intervention (PCI)- Procedure to treat acute MI. Fibrinolytics may be placed to dissolve clots.

Percutaneous transluminal coronary angioplasty (PTCA)- Procedure used to place stents to maintain the patency of an artery.

Transesophageal echocardiography (TEE)- A diagnostic procedure to assess ventricular and valve function, cardiac structures, blood flow velocity and other cardiac parameters.

Valve replacement- The new valve can be made from many different types of materials and from different doners- Pig, horse, human, cow, Dacron, or metal. Patients with new valves may be asked to eat a diet low in calcium to avoid build up on new valve.

Your facility may require nurses to be ACLS certified. In ACLS, you will learn several abnormal heart rhythms and treatment for each. Below are some examples of abnormal heart rhythms.

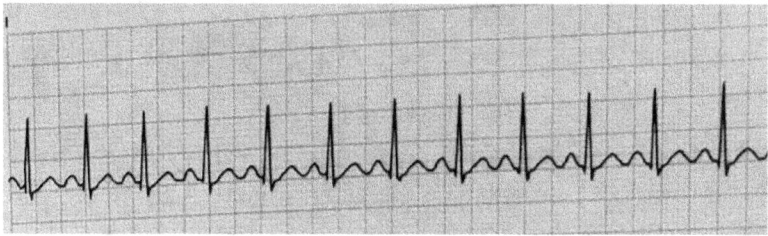

Sinus tachycardia

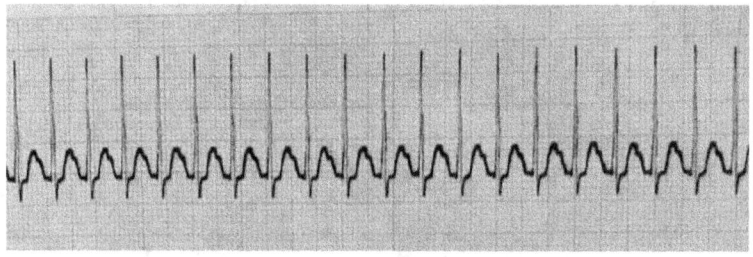

Supraventricular tachycardia

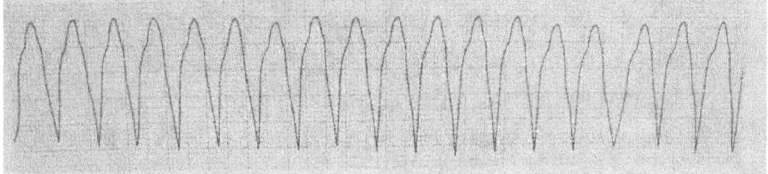

Monomorphic ventricular tachycardia

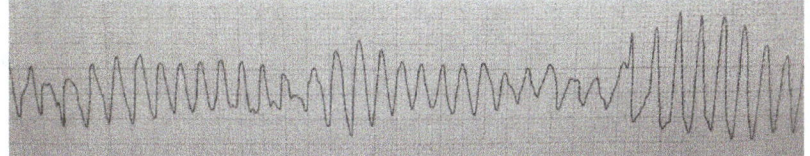

Torsade de Pointes is a type of polymorphic ventricular tachycardia.

Christmas day is the most common day of the year to have a heart attack. Most heart attacks happen on a Monday.

Endocrine

Hormones

- **Adrenocortical-** Hyposecretion can cause Addison's disease, a condition where insufficient glucose is synthesized. The body may not deal well with stress and may lead to shock due to the sodium loss in urine. Hypersecretion can cause Cushing's disease. Patients may present with edema in the face, which may be described as a "Moon face." The condition also includes increased blood glucose and a decreased immune response.

- **Insulin-** A lack of insulin can cause diabetes mellitus. An excess of insulin causes hypoglycemia.

- **Parathyroid-** hyposecretion can cause spasms and death. Hypersecretion can cause kidney stones and weak bones.

- **Thyroid-** A lack of thyroid hormone can cause bradycardia, myxedema, and a decrease in the basal metabolic rate. Hypersecretion can cause tachycardia, weight loss, and basal metabolic rate increase.

Glossary:

Chvostek's sign- Twitching of the facial muscles in response to tapping the face. Sign of hypocalcemia.

Kussmaul's breathing- Rapid, deep breathing at a consistent rhythm. It is associated with patients who have diabetes with ketoacidosis.

Trousseau's sign- A blood pressure cuff or tourniquet is placed on the patient. The sign is positive and indicates hypocalcemia when the patient demonstrates a carpopedal spasm.

Thyroid- Located in the anterior neck with the right lobe below the larynx and the left lobe beside the trachea. The isthmus is the middle section which is located at the base of the neck between the second and fourth tracheal rings. Hormones are produced that regulate metabolism and growth.

Postoperative care includes:

- Encouraging the patient to refrain from speaking to rest the vocal cords.
- Monito the neck dressing for drainage,
- Monitor airway.
- To assess for nerve damage, have the patient say "E"
- Watch for symptoms of hypocalcemia.

Hyperthyroid	Hypothyroid
Low or high blood pressure	Puffy eyes
Tachycardia	Bradycardia
Weight loss	Weight gain
Increased peristalsis	Constipation
Diaphoresis	Dry skin
Heat intolerance	Cold intolerance
Hyperactive emotions	Inability to concentrate
Insomnia	Fatigue
TSH decreased	TSH increased

Conditions that are seen with hyper and hypothyroid
Infertility
High blood pressure
Goiter
Hoarseness, difficulty swallowing

Parathyroid- Four small glands located behind the thyroid. Parathyroid hormone (PTH) and vitamin D regulate calcium and phosphorus. Rising serum calcium levels inhibit PTH. PTH release is dependent on normal serum magnesium levels.

Pituitary gland- Located at the base of the skull. Hormones include human growth hormone,

122

ACTH, thyroid-stimulating, luteinizing, prolactin, and ADH. Postoperative care includes monitoring the respiratory and oxygenation status, managing secretions, calcium levels, Chvostek's sign, and surgical site hematoma.

Adrenal glands- Located on the medial aspect of the superior pole of each kidney. Responsible for carbohydrate and protein metabolism, controls blood pressure by regulating sodium and water reabsorption, and has anti-inflammatory effects. A hyposecretion of cortisol and aldosterone causes Addison's disease. Cushing's syndrome is caused by hypersecretion of corticosteroids. An overproduction of catecholamines causes Pheochromocytoma.

Signs of hypocalcemia-

- Carpopedal spasms
- Convulsions
- Chvostek's sign- Face spasm when the facial nerve is tapped.
- Muscle cramps
- Paresthesia
- Trousseau sign- Blood pressure cuff inflated will induce muscle spasms in the hand and forearm.

Diabetes- Diabetic patients are at a higher risk for surgical and anesthetic complications. Regional blocks may be performed to lessen the risks of anesthesia.

Hypoglycemia	Hyperglycemia
Shakiness	Polydipsia
Diaphoresis	Skin warm and dry
Confusion	Polyphagia
Seizures	Tall, peaked T waves on EKG
Irritability	Fruity breath
	Polyuria
	Kussmaul's respiration

Hypo and hyperglycemia
Decreased level of consciousness
Tachycardia

Gastrointestinal

Glossary-

Adhesions- Scar tissue that connects two normally separate surfaces. It can be a fibrous band. It can cause obstructions or malfunctions of organs.

Dysphagia- Difficulty swallowing

Odynophagia- Painful swallowing

Omphalocele- A congenital disability seen in infants. This rare condition may be associated with other conditions. A defect in the periumbilical wall may cause a sac containing the small and /or large bowel.

Peristalsis- Constriction and relaxation of the intestine to create a wave-like action that propels the contents through the GI tract.

Anatomy:

Esophagus

The GI tract begins with the mouth which is attached to the esophagus by the pharynx. Located posterior to the trachea. There are three layers- the mucosa, submucosa, and the muscularis. The lower esophageal sphincter controls the passage of food into the stomach.

Stomach

Initiates digestion through chemical and mechanical means.

Small Intestine

The stomach's pyloric sphincter empties into the duodenum, which continues into the jejunum and then into the ilium. The small intestine is responsible for digestion, absorption, and immunologic functions and provides secretions and barriers to infections.

Large Intestine

The ileocecal valve from the small intestine connects with the cecum, where the vermiform appendix is located. The ascending colon is connected to the cecum, which passes up the right side of the abdomen. The transverse colon crosses the abdomen from right to left connecting to the descending colon. The sigmoid colon follows and is attached to the rectum. The anal canal connects to the anus.

Liver

The liver detoxifies chemicals, makes bile, and stores energy. The liver or liver lobs may be removed for cancer or trauma. Post-op care for a patient with hepatic lobectomy includes monitoring for bleeding, electrolyte imbalance, and liver or kidney failure. Liver transplants may be performed using a liver from a cadaver or a partial liver from a living relative.

Patients recovering from liver procedures should be watched for bleeding. Positioning the patient is important after certain procedures, such as a liver biopsy, where the patient is kept on the right side for two hours.

Gallbladder

The gallbladder is located on the underside of the right lobe of the liver. When certain types of food enter the duodenum, bile is released from the gallbladder. Bile consists of cholesterol, inorganic salts, phospholipids, pigments, bile acids, and water. Cholelithiasis is the presence of stones. Cholecystitis is caused by duct obstruction from impacted gallstones, infection, or injury due to trauma. Signs and symptoms of affected gallbladder include:

- Pain in abdomen
- Nausea and vomiting
- Intolerance to certain foods- fats
- Jaundice
- Fever

Laparoscopic or open cholecystectomy may be performed for removal of the gallbladder. Laparoscopic cholecystectomy, or lap chole, can be done with three or four small abdominal puncture sites. The lap chole is often less painful than an open one but may take longer. The benefits of a lap chole vs. open include a shorter recovery time and fewer complications. Surgery may start out laparoscopic but turn into open surgery if needed.

Post-operative care includes pain assessment with instructions to the patient to be aware that pain in the shoulder is normal due to the CO_2 gas used to inflate the abdomen during laparoscopic surgery.

Pancreas

Produces insulin and digestive enzymes. The pancreas may be removed to treat cancer, necrosis, or trauma. A pancreas transplant may be performed to treat diabetes.

Pancreaticoduodenectomy- Whipple's procedure- is used to treat cancer on the head of the pancreas. The proximal portion of the pancreas, lower portion of the stomach, gallbladder, and common bile duct are removed.

Postoperative care includes managing nausea and vomiting, monitoring fluid volumes, possible drains care, preventing DVT, and encouraging cough and deep breathing to prevent respiratory compromise. The surgeon may leave strict orders not to manipulate the NG tube. The patient's diet may be slowly advanced. Pain control is important. The patient may have a PCA or an epidural pain pump.

Monitor for respiratory compromise in case of overmedication and sedation from pain medications.

Conditions and diseases:

Crohn's disease may affect any part of the GI tract but is most commonly found in the terminal ileum. Crohn's is a transmural submucosal inflammatory condition.

Diverticula- Outpouchings of one or more layers of the wall of the GI tract.

Diverticulosis- Uncomplicated diverticular disease.

Diverticulitis- Inflammation of the diverticulum, commonly found in the sigmoid colon. It can lead to rupture or obstruction.

Gastroesophageal reflux disease (GERD)- A reflux of gastric acid into the esophagus. It can cause heartburn, dysphagia, or respiratory conditions.

Hemorrhoid- A vascular mass in the anal canal.

Hiatal hernia- A condition where part of the stomach protrudes through the diaphragm into the thoracic cavity.

Intussusception- A condition where the bowel telescopes onto itself.

Mallory-Weiss Tear- Mucosal tear at the gastroesophageal junction. It can be caused by vomiting, trauma, childbirth, or after a scope procedure.

Peptic ulcer disease- May be caused by Helicobacter pylori (H. pylori), stress, medications, and trauma. It can lead to bleeding or perforations. Most are found in the duodenum.

Polyps- Tissue masses that protrude into the lumen of the bowel. Most are asymptomatic. Some patients may experience bleeding. Removal of polyps can decrease the occurrence of cancer.

Short bowel syndrome- May be caused by the removal of part of the small bowel surgically or from genetic causes. Causes malabsorption of nutrients and fluids.

Varices can occur in the GI tract but are most commonly found in the submucosal veins of the distal esophagus, stomach, and hemorrhoidal plexus. It may be associated with portal hypertension due to alcoholic cirrhosis.

Procedures and surgery:

Barium swallow- Imaging study to examine the upper GI tract- throat, esophagus, stomach, and duodenum.

Cholangiogram- Visualizes the structure of the bile ducts and the gallbladder. It may be performed during cholecystectomy.

Colectomy- Removal of all or part of the colon commonly done for patients with cancer, trauma, and necrosis. The patient may require a colostomy.

Colonoscopy- A scope is used to visualize the lower GI tract. Tissues may be biopsied.

Colostomy- A fistula is created to combine the colon with the abdominal wall. It may be temporary or permanent. The stoma should be pink and moist.

Endoscopic Retrograde Cholangiopancreatography (ERCP)- Uses endoscopy and radiologic techniques to visualize biliary and pancreatic ducts.

Esophagogastroduodenoscopy (EGD)- A flexible scope is passed through the GI tract to visualize structures and take biopsies. The nurse should assist with helping the patient maintain a patent airway by assisting with positioning and suctioning.

Esophagoscopy- Can be combined with a collection of specimens for biopsy. It can be used to determine anatomical abnormalities.

Gastrectomy- Removal of all or a portion of the stomach. It may be done for cancer treatment.

o   Billroth 1- First section of duodenum sewn to the remaining section of the stomach after stomach section removal.
o   Billroth 2- The first section of the duodenum is sewn shut with a loop of jejunum sewn to the remaining stomach section.
o   Roux-en-Y gastrojejunostomy- Performed after total gastrectomy as a reconstruction procedure of the stomach.

Hernia repair- Classified according to location. Displacement of viscus- usually bowel- through an opening, either congenital or created. It may be an elective surgery or emergent if strangulation and necrosis have occurred. It may be performed open or laparoscopically. Watch for scrotal swelling after inguinal hernia repair, which may indicate bleeding. Some types of hernia:

- o Epigastric
- o Incisional
- o Inguinal
- o Femoral
- o Umbilical
- o Ventral

Laparotomy- A procedure that opens the abdominal wall to the peritoneal cavity. Not as common as in the past due to laparoscopic and robotic techniques. It may be done for large tumors or for trauma.

If infection or bowel spillage occurs, the patient may be left with the surgical wound open. The wound may be packed, or a negative pressure vacuum may be placed. The nurse should monitor the vacuum to ensure the battery is charged, the device is plugged in, and the canister for collection is not full.

Nissen fundoplication- To treat GERD. A portion of the stomach is wrapped around the distal esophagus. Watch for aspiration postoperatively.

Percutaneous Endoscopic Gastrostomy (PEG)- A tube may be inserted surgically into the stomach for feeding purposes.

Sigmoidoscopy- Less invasive than a colonoscopy when an examination of only the sigmoid colon is needed.

Trans jugular intrahepatic portosystemic shunt (TIPS)- Procedure for portal hypertension patients. A needle is advanced from a hepatic vein to a portal branch. A stent is placed.

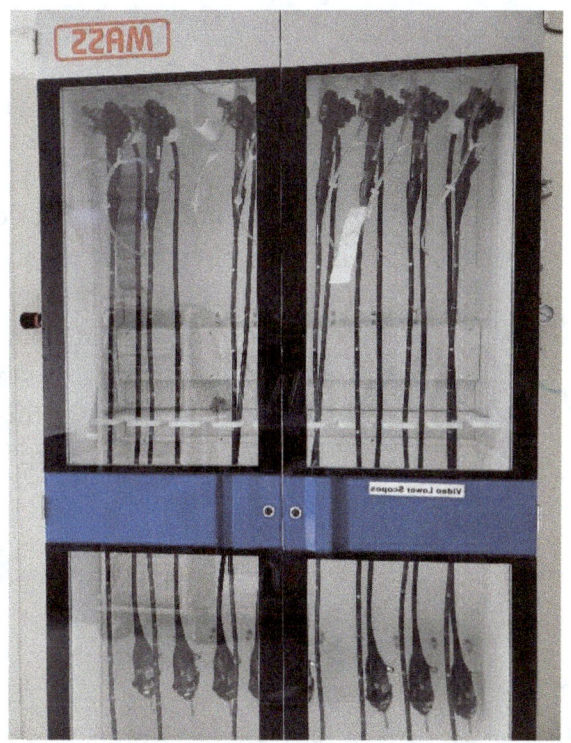

A storage cabinet with GI scopes

General post-op care for GI patients

- Gastric and colonic peristalsis may not be present for up to five days post-op.

- Nasogastric tubes may be placed. Check the orders from the surgeon to determine how much suction, if any, is needed.

- Laparoscopic surgery may involve inflating the abdomen with gas to allow visualization. The gas tends to irritate the diaphragm and cause referred shoulder pain for the patient. The patient cannot "Fart it out." The pain will go away on its own. Warn the patient of this to prevent unpleasant surprises when the patient gets home.

- Drains are common. Follow the surgeon's orders for suction and irrigation.

- Occasionally a patient will accidentally fall down in the shower and land on an object that will need to be removed from the rectum under anesthesia. Most of these objects can be removed through the same route they went in. However, if the object punctures the rectum or if the surgeon cannot get the object out, the patient

may need open abdominal surgery
and possibly a colostomy.

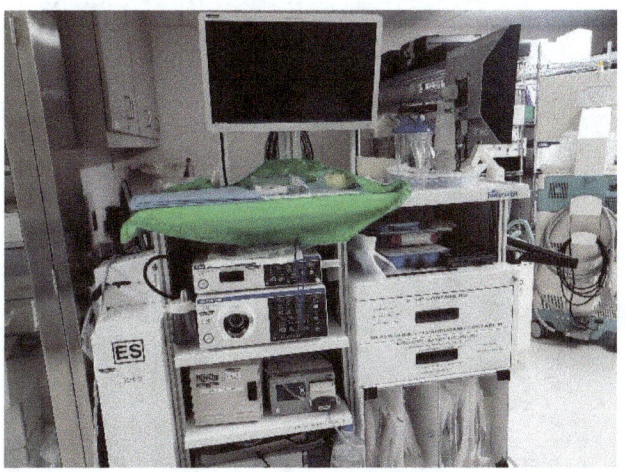

A GI scope cart ready to go.

Incision locations:

1-Kocher incision- For gallbladder surgery

2- Upper midline

3- McBurney incision- appendix

4- Lower abdominal incision

5- Inguinal

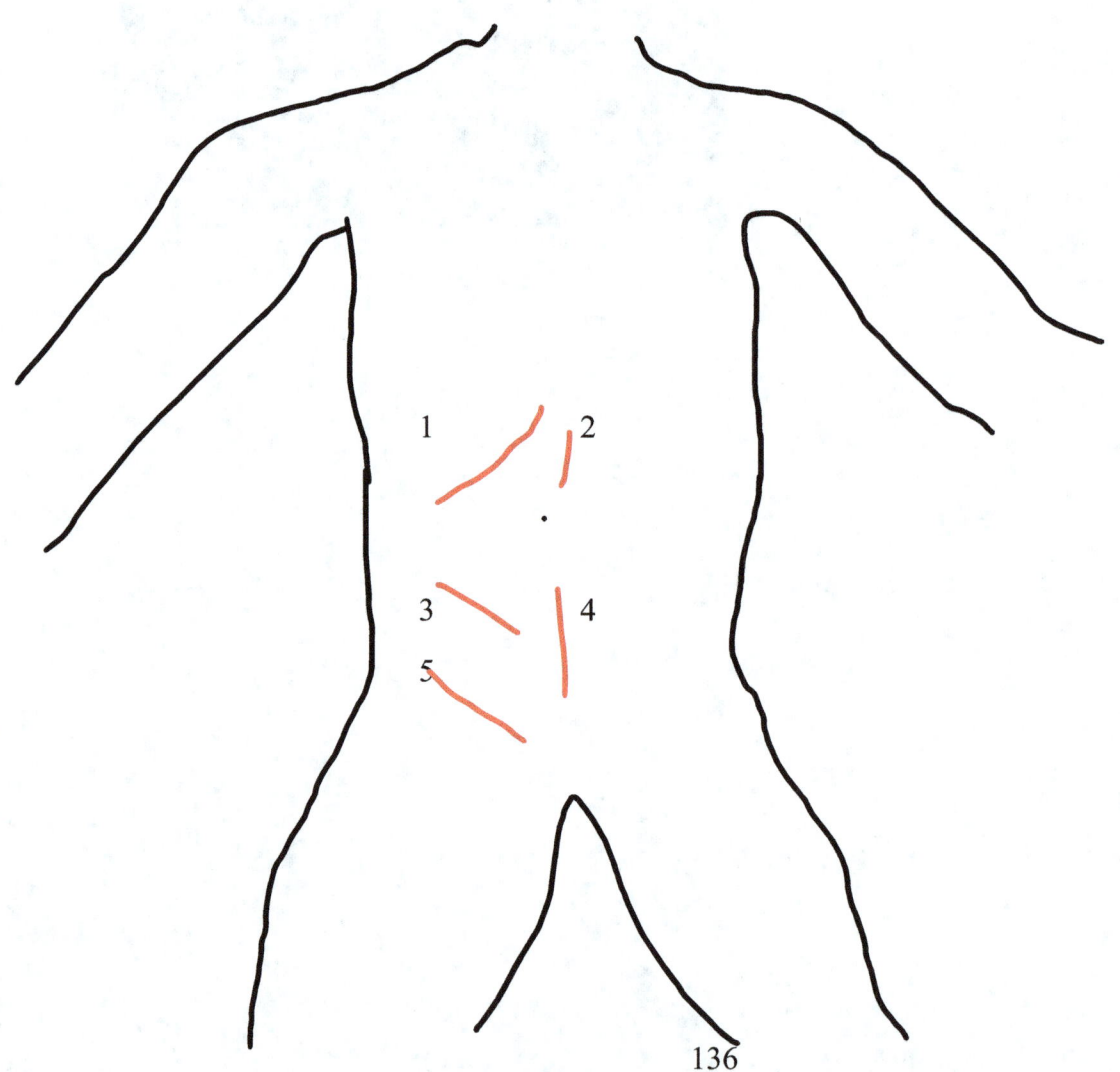

genitourinary

Glossary-

Enuresis- Incontinence of urine, often during sleep.

Hematuria- Blood in the urine.

Anatomy-

Adrenal glands: Located on each kidney.

Secrete hormones-

o Glucocorticoid: cortisol- released during physiologic or emotional stress. It Stimulates glucose, fat, and protein catabolism and is anti-inflammatory.

o Mineralocorticoid: Aldosterone- renin-angiotensin-aldosterone stimulated release. Promotes sodium reabsorption and excretion of potassium. The primary mechanism for potassium secretion.

o Epinephrine and norepinephrine- fight-or-flight response increases heart rate and blood pressure.

The sympathetic nervous system uses neurotransmitters.

Addison's disease- Adrenal insufficiency caused by the destruction of the adrenal cortex from autoimmune disease. May requires hormone replacement therapy. It may cause an adrenal crisis which is a life-threatening emergency. Give IV fluids and steroids.

Cushing's disease- Caused by excessive serum cortisol from an overproduction of adrenocorticotropic hormone- ACTH, cancer, or in patients receiving steroids. Patients may have weakness, especially in the quadriceps, "moon face," "buffalo hump," striae on thighs and abdomen, poor skin turgor, sleep disturbances, slow wound healing, osteoporosis, will easily bruise, or renal calculi. Treatment may include bilateral adrenalectomy or transsphenoidal hypophysectomy.

Kidney- Parenchyma is the functional part of the kidney. This contains approximately 1.2 million nephrons, the kidney's functional units. A patient only needs one kidney to have adequate renal function.

Normal urine output is 0.5-1.0 ML/KG/HR. Oliguria is the patient has less than 30 Ml/HR, 100 ML/4 HR, or 400-500 ML/ 24HR. Polyuria is increased urine production- over 3000 ML/ 24 HR. Specific gravity is usually less than 1.003 with polyuria. Polyuria can be caused by a pituitary tumor or pituitary manipulation or in a diabetic patient with increased blood sugar.

A patient with chronic renal failure should not be given Lactated Ringers as it may cause acidosis. Give these patients normal saline or 5% dextrose instead.

Postoperatively, patients should be monitored for urine output, hydration status, and prevention of infection. For surgeries involving the removal of a kidney or kidney transplant, avoid toxic medications to prevent harm to the remaining kidney. A central venous pressure monitor may be in place to help maintain hydration.

AV shunt- May be placed in the wrist, forearm, or upper arm. Post-operative care includes auscultating for bruit and palpating for a pulse every 15 minutes in the recovery room, phase 1. Help the patient keep the arm extended and elevated to prevent swelling. Include in the post-operative instructions to keep the arm elevated for 24 hours at home.

The kidneys filter approximately 180 liters of plasma in a day. All plasma is filtered about 60 times a day.

Hemorrhage, heart failure, and dehydration are triggers for renin to be released. Renin converts plasma protein angiotensin to angiotensin 1. Angiotensin converting enzyme converts to angiotensin 2. Angiotensin 2 is a vasoconstrictor and increases blood pressure.

Prostaglandin from the renal medulla modulates renin release. Prostaglandin affects urine concentration.

Aldosterone is released from the adrenal cortex. Decreased sodium and increased potassium may cause the release of aldosterone, which will cause the kidney to absorb more sodium and excrete more potassium. This can help prevent acidosis.

The kidney secretes erythropoietin to stimulate the production of red blood cells.

Antidiuretic hormone- vasopressin- is secreted by the pituitary gland to increase water reabsorption and decrease urine output when water is lost.

See the vascular section for more information on fistula creation for dialysis.

Female anatomy-

Bartholin's gland- Located in the inner aspect of the labia minora within the vagina. Supplements lubrication. Occlusion of the gland can cause cysts and infections.

Skene's gland- Located on the floor or urethra inside the meatus. Aids in lubrication of the vagina.

Three layers of the uterus:

o Perimetrium- Outer layer
o Myometrium- Middle muscular wall.
o Endometrium- Inner layer

Male anatomy:

Prostate gland- Contributes to seminal fluid, contracts during ejaculation, and transports sperm to ejaculate. Shaped like a donut, it surrounds the urethra. It contains five lobes or zones; the peripheral zone is the most common origination of prostate cancers.

Cowper's glands- pea-size glands that secrete mucous during ejaculation, located on each side of the posterior urethra.

Seminal vesicles- membranous pouches located under the base of the bladder and above the prostate gland. Forms ejaculatory duct by joining vas deferens.

Spermatic cord- Located bilaterally to testes through the inguinal canal to the internal inguinal ring. Contains vas deferens, spermatic arteries, and autonomic nerves.

Conditions and diseases:

Balanoposthitis- Inflamed penis and mucous membranes. The patient may have purulent drainage from the penis. It may require circumcision.

Cryptorchidism- Undescended testes that may cause sterility if not corrected by 1 to 2 years.

Epispadias- Absence of dorsal urethral wall.

Hydrocele- A collection of fluid in the scrotal sac that may compromise the blood supply to the testicles.

Hypospadias- The opening of the urethral meatus is not at the tip of the penis. It may require surgical intervention.

Phimosis- A condition where the foreskin is unretractable over the penis. The patient may need a circumcision.

Paraphimosis- A condition where the foreskin is retracted and may cause swelling or dry gangrene. Circumcision may be needed.

Spermatocele- Obstruction of sperm carrying tubular system causes an intrascrotal cyst. Common after vasectomy.

Testicular torsion- Testicular blood supply is compromised; the patient typically needs emergency surgery to correct it before permanent damage occurs.

Varicocele- Venous backflow causes veins of the spermatic cord to become engorged.

Procedures:

Post-op care includes monitoring for bleeding, urinary retention, and fluid and electrolyte balances. The patient should be watched for hyponatremia if a large amount of irrigant was used. Education may include home care of foleys or drains and infection prevention. The patient may have a fear of cancer diagnosis, incontinence, or sexual dysfunction, depending on the procedure.

A patient may need continuous bladder irrigation. This is done using a three-way foley. The irrigant is infused into the bladder through one port. Another port is used to inflate the balloon. The third port empties the urine and irrigant from the bladder. These patients need to be monitored closely to prevent the urine from becoming too red with clots. The bladder must not be allowed to develop clots that may occlude the urine flow. A surgeon may order the patient to have traction on a Foley catheter. Monitor bleed.

Bladder neck suspension- Performed to correct urinary incontinence.

Circumcision- Commonly done on adults to remove the constricting foreskin.

Cystogram- The installation of dye visualizes the bladder via cystoscopy or catheterization.

Cystoscopy- A flexible or rigid scope is placed through the urethra to examine the bladder, urethra, prostate, and ureters. Biopsies may be taken, medication such as chemotherapy may be instilled, or calculi may be removed.

Extracorporeal shock wave lithotripsy- External shock waves are directed at the patient's kidney to help break up calculi. The surgeon may ask the patient to strain their urine at home and bring any stones into the follow-up appointment. This is a noninvasive process but may leave a hematoma at the site.

Hypospadias/ urethroplasty- Commonly done on children. Repositioning of the urethral meatus or meatal reconstruction.

Intravenous pyelogram- Contrast dye is given intravenously to enable visualization of the urinary system.

Orchidopexy- Performed for patients with undescended testis or for testicular torsion to prevent a recurrence. Commonly performed on children.

Orchiectomy- Removal of the testis. Concern for cardiac dysrhythmia from traction on the spermatic cord.

Penectomy- Partial or total removal of the penis. It may be done for cancer or trauma. Complications include sloughing of skin and loss of ability to urinate.

Prostatectomy- May be performed open, laparoscopy, or robotic. May be located retropubic, perineal, or suprapubic.

Retrograde pyelogram- Used for direct vision and fluoroscopic views of ureters and kidneys through cystoscopy and radiographic dye.

Transurethral resection of bladder tumor or bladder neck- Cystoscopy procedure. Monitor the patient's emotional condition and possible diagnosis of cancer.

Transurethral resection of the prostate (TURP)- A prostatectomy. Performed for BPH. A laser may be used.

Gynecological

Some facilities separate gynecological surgeries; other facilities combine GYN surgeries with everything else. As a recovery room nurse, you may need to recover cesarian section patients or other procedures such as dilation, curettage, or tubal ligations. In your facility, you may not ever see these types of patients. If you are planning on sitting for a certification exam such as CAPA or CPAN, you may need to know the basics.

Pregnancy

- Increased cardiac output- 30 to 50%
- Increased HR
- Increased breathing and increased tidal volume.
- Increased blood glucose
- Decreased gastric motility- can increase the risk of aspiration.
- Pregnant women are in a state of compensated respiratory alkalemia.
- Pregnancy risks and considerations for surgery:

o Preeclampsia- Magnesium is given IV to prevent seizures. Magnesium may cause an increased risk of respiratory depression.

o Post-op cesarean delivery, the uterus should be firm and midline. Oxytocin increases uterine contractions and can stop bleeding.

o Post-delivery, the lochia should have clots and be dark- rubra- or bright red. The absence of clots could indicate disseminated intravascular coagulation, DIC.

o Post-partum hemorrhage is considered to be more than 500 ML of blood. The first sign of hemorrhagic shock in these patients may be mild tachycardia.

o Assess fetal heart tones during and/or after surgery.

o Decreased amounts of anesthetic drugs may be used.

o Increased risk of aspiration and failed intubation due to anatomical changes due to pregnancy.

o Halogenated gases decrease uterine resting tone, uterine muscle tension, and spontaneous uterine activity, nitrous oxide has no significant effect on uterine tone, and ketamine increases uterine resting tone.

o Keep a wedge under the patient during surgery to prevent aorta compression, and lay the patient on the left side if possible.

Abortion terms- Abortion is a term that implies the death of a fetus or removal of a fetus from a uterus. Laypeople often use the term miscarriage to describe a fetal death. The term abortion is often used as a term for birth control or the intentional death of a fetus. Be careful with the terminology around patients who may be grieving; the word abortion may not be taken well by a woman who had an unwanted loss of her fetus.

- Incomplete- Products of conception are left behind in the uterus after fetal death.
- Missed- The fetus died before 20 weeks gestation, and products of conception have remained.
- Therapeutic- Performed by medical care provider when the mother's mental or physical health is at risk.
- Spontaneous- This also means miscarriage.

With the loss of the pregnancy, the patient may need emotional support. The patient may be grieving the loss of the child she was expecting but may be told by well-meaning friends and family that she was not really pregnant anyway (as in a hydatidiform mole) or that she is young, she can have more, or it is God's will or other statements that will possibly inadvertently make her feel worse. Just tell her you are sorry and answer any questions she may have. Some facilities have chaplains who can talk to the patient and family. This might make them feel like they are supported. The chaplains have been trained to help people who are grieving.

Complications during pregnancy:

Abrupto placenta – The placenta separates partially or totally prematurely. It may cause hemorrhage.

Bicornuate uterus- Most commonly, an abnormally shaped uterus with two "horns" near the top.

Chronic hypertension- Hypertension is diagnosed before the 20th week of pregnancy and may last more than 12 weeks after delivery.

DIC- Disseminated intravascular coagulation- Abnormal clotting throughout the body. At a higher risk if experiencing preeclampsia, HELLP, or abrupto placentae.

Ectopic pregnancy- A pregnancy outside of the uterus, usually in the fallopian tube. If the fallopian tube ruptures, the patient may hemorrhage to death.

Preeclampsia- Reduced organ perfusion in pregnancy due to hypertension. Other features include proteinuria, visual disturbances, and hepatic involvement.

Eclampsia-Patient may experience seizures or coma. Give magnesium to help control seizures.

HELLP- Hemolysis, elevated liver enzymes, low platelets. A form of severe pre-eclampsia.

Hydatidiform mole- Multiple cysts that cause rapid uterine growth. The patient has a hemorrhage risk. The patient shows signs and symptoms of pregnancy.

Intrahepatic cholestasis- A liver disorder that is characterized by a buildup of bile that can cause itching.

Post-partum hemorrhage- loss of greater than 500 ml of blood. It may be caused by uterine atony or lacerations.

Placenta previa- The placenta is implanted in the lower uterine segment. It may cause hemorrhage.

Uterine inversion- The uterus turns inside out after delivery. Potentially life-threatening. The uterus may be able to be replaced. Watch for shock and hemorrhage.

Procedures during pregnancy:

Cerclage- Attempt to stop a miscarriage. A stitch is placed to help keep the cervix closed.

Dilation and curettage/ evacuation- Removal of materials from the uterus. A curet is a spoon-shaped instrument. This may be done after a missed or incomplete abortion.

Spinal anesthesia-Anatomical changes during pregnancy have implications for spinal anesthesia. The patient's increased blood volume and pressure of the uterus on the vena cava may lead to the engorgement of epidural veins. There is an increased risk of intravascular injections and catheter migration into epidural veins.

Postoperative care-

Noncomplicated vaginal birth- Watch for orthostatic hypotension and hemorrhage. Fundus should be firm and midline at the level of the umbilicus for the first 24 hours; monitor for bladder distention.

Cesarean section- Treat as any abdominal surgery with additional complications as seen with vaginal birth.

Medications commonly used in obstetrics

- Alprostadil (Prostin)- Used to increase uterine contractions.

- Labetalol- Anti-hypertensive.

- Magnesium sulfate- Used to treat neuromuscular and CNS irritability. Used for patients experiencing pre-eclampsia and inhibits preterm contractions. Potential complications include respiratory depression and cardiovascular collapse. Calcium gluconate is the antidote.

- Oxytocin- Increases uterine contractions.

- Pitocin- Used for postpartum bleeding and to stimulate milk ejection. It may cause hypotension if not properly diluted.

- RhoGAM- Depresses immune response. Given to women after exposure to Rh-positive blood.

- Tocolytics- Relaxes smooth muscle and inhibits preterm labor and bronchospasms. It may cause tremors and anxiety.

Anatomy:

Labia majora- Outer vulval lips

Labia minora- Inner vulval lips

Clitoris- Small organ below the arch of the mons pubis

Bartholin's gland- Located in the inner aspect of the labia minora within the vagina.

Supplements lubrication. Occlusion of the gland can cause cysts and infections. A bartholinectomy may be performed to facilitate drainage.

Skene's gland- Located on the floor or urethra inside the meatus. Aids in lubrication of the vagina.

Hymen- Thin membrane that partially covers the vaginal orifice.

Fallopian tubes- Carry ova into the uterus.

Three layers of the uterus:

- Perimetrium- Outer layer
- Myometrium- Middle muscular wall.
- Endometrium- Inner layer

Ovaries- Produce ova, estrogen, progesterone.

Ligaments of the uterus- Hold the uterus in place, eight in total.

- Two cardinal
- Two lateral or broad
- Two uterosacral
- Two round

Conditions:

Imperforated hymen- Completely closed hymen. A hymenectomy may be performed to enlarge the vaginal opening.

Procedures:

Surgery is often completed with the patient in the lithotomy position. This position requires the patient to have their legs in stirrups. This position has the potential to cause nerve damage in the legs or back. Caution should be taken to prevent the patient's fingers from being crushed when the table bottom is lowered. When lowering the patient's legs, use two staff members to lower both legs at the same time to prevent nerve damage.

Common postop complaints from patients include cramping or loss of emotional control. The patient may be crying but does not know why. Provide emotional comfort and reassure them they can cry; it is normal. Give a heating pad and pain medications, and let the patient lay in a position of comfort if able.

It is common for gyn procedures to have post-op bleeding from the vagina. The most common post-op instructions for procedures include teaching that bleeding is normal, but if the patient soaks a peri pad in an hour, to notify the provider. The discharge should not smell bad, be green or other strange colors, and should gradually subside. If there are signs of infection, the provider should be notified.

Anterior colporrhaphy- Removal of excess posterior vaginal tissue to tighten the vaginal wall.

Cervical conization and colposcopy- Removal of a cone of tissue from the cervix to diagnose infection or cancer.

Endometrial ablation- Procedure to dysfunctional uterine bleeding. The uterine lining is "burned" with a laser, electricity, or other device to slow or stop bleeding. The patient will be infertile after the procedure.

Hysterectomy- Removal of the uterus and possibly the fallopian tubes. The ovaries may be removed as well, depending on the reason for the procedure, such as cancer. The procedure may be performed vaginally, laparoscopically, or through an open procedure.

Hysteroscopy- An endoscopic procedure to look inside the uterus. Biopsies may be taken, polyps may be removed, and foreign bodies may be placed or removed, such as IUDs, or for diagnosis. Complications may occur due to the large amount of irrigation used. Hyponatremia, hypoproteinemia, or circulatory overload may occur. Fluids such as saline, glycine, or dextran may be used.

Loop electrosurgical excision procedure (LEEP)- Removes intact tissue for diagnostics.

Oophorectomy- Removal of the ovary.

Tension-free vaginal tape (TVT)- Procedure to correct stress incontinence A mesh tape is placed under the mid urethra. The patient may need to self-catheterize after the procedure.

Tubal ligation- Procedure is done for female sterilization. The fallopian tubes may be cut and cauterized, removed completely, clipped with filshie clips, or other devices may be placed to occlude the tubes.

Mental Health

Patients with cognitive deficits from birth, mental health issues such as schizophrenia, or conditions such as post-traumatic stress may present to the surgical department. Patients may also be in a mental health crisis and have an acute surgical emergency concurrently, such as appendicitis. Other patients may be admitted for treatments such as ECT- electroconvulsive therapy which is used to treat depression.

Patients may have communication difficulties and may need assistive devices. If a patient is severely depressed, they may not make eye contact or speak to you.

Some patients may be scared or paranoid. These patients should be approached slowly with no sudden movements. Do not whisper or talk near the patient without including them in the conversation. Do not touch the patient without giving a warning and receiving permission. If the patient is having hallucinations, do not feed into the hallucination or try to argue with the patient.

Electroconvulsive therapy (ECT)-
Performed on patients who have severe depression. Commonly known as shock therapy. A certain movie from the 70s features an awesome nurse in a psychiatric hospital that demonstrates this. Thankfully ECTs are much nicer these days.

The patient is seen by a psychiatrist who determines whether the patient may benefit from the procedure. The patient is then admitted to a facility that performs ECTs. The patient is given general anesthesia. A tourniquet is placed on the patient's ankle. A paralytic is given. The electrodes are placed on the patient to give a shock to cause a seizure in the patient's brain. The paralytic has not been able to enter the patient's foot due to the tourniquet, so the foot will move during the seizure. The rest of the body does not. The patient is allowed to wake up and recover from anesthesia.

Treatments usually occur two to three times a week for many weeks. I have personally cared for patients receiving this type of therapy. It works well for some. For others, there is less or no effect.

Neuro and Spine

Anatomy and physiology

The neuron is the basic structural unit of the central nervous system. The neuron has three main parts- the cell body, the axon, and the dendrite.

The **nerve cell** receives and conducts impulses. The afferent, or sensory, neurons conduct impulses from receptors to the central nervous system, while the efferent or motor neurons conduct impulses from the central nervous system to effector organs.

The axon is the longest process and conducts impulses away from the cell body. The axon may be myelinated, which is insulated or unmyelinated. '

The dendrites are short processes with multiple projections that conduct impulses toward the cell body and can receive information.

Synapse- A junction between two nerve cells.

Afferent- Term used to describe sensory impulses being carried toward the brain.

Efferent- The term describes sensory impulses carried away from the brain.

Autonomic nervous system- Regulates the unconscious body functions such as heart rate, digestion, and temperature.

Sympathetic nervous system- Responsible for the fight or flight response.

Chemical transmissions:

- Neurotransmitters- Made from protein, stimulate, facilitate, or inhibit impulse transmission.
    - Adrenergic- dopamine, norepinephrine, epinephrine
    - Cholinergic- acetylcholine
    - Serotonin
    - Histamine

Meninges protect the brain and spinal cord and support underlying structures. Layers from Inner to Outer:

- Pia mater- one cell thick, in direct contact with the brain.
- Arachnoid membrane- separated from dura mater by subdural space.
- Dura mater- double layer with folds. Divides cranial vault into left and right hemispheres, occipital and temporal lobes.

Subdural space is a potential space that is located below the dura and above the arachnoid. The

158

subarachnoid space contains the cerebral spinal fluid, the arteries, and the veins. The arterial system is two systems, anterior and posterior, that combine to form the circle of Willis.

- Anterior arterial circulation includes:
    - The common carotid branches into the external and internal carotid arteries
    - The anterior cerebral artery supplies the medial surfaces of the frontal and parietal lobes.
    - Anterior communicating artery
    - The middle cerebral artery is the large branch of the internal carotid artery and supplies two-thirds of the lateral surface of cerebral hemispheres.

- Posterior arterial circulation
    - Vertebral arteries are paired arteries that arise from the subclavian artery that enters the cranial vault through the foramen magnum. These branches supply the spinal cord, the underside of the cerebellum, the medulla, and the choroid plexus of the fourth ventricle. The paired arteries merge to form the basilar artery, which branches into the posterior cerebral arteries that supply the posterior fossa.
    - The posterior cerebral artery supplies the brainstem, occipital lobe, and inferior and medial surfaces of the temporal lobe.

The cerebral spinal fluid (CSF) cushions and carries nutrients to the brain. Most CSF is formed in the lateral ventricle by the choroid plexus. Approximately 500 ml per day of CSF is produced, with 150 ml in the system at a time. Four fluid-filled cavities- ventricles- circulate CSF through all four ventricles, the spinal canal, and the subarachnoid space. CSF is clear, colorless, and odorless. CSF contains:

- Chloride 120- 130 mcg/L
- Glucose- 50 to 75 mg/dl
- PH- 7.35-7.40
- Protein 15 to 45 mg/dl
- WBC- 0-5/ mm
- No RBC

The brain's outermost layer is the cerebral cortex, which is made up of gray matter. The gyri are the raised projections of the brain, and the sulci are the grooves. The left side is involved with language, math, and reasoning. The right involves the creative aspect and visual-spatial tasks. The brain is divided into lobes:

- Two frontal lobes control voluntary and fine motor movement. This lobe contains memory, emotions, and complex functions.
- Two parietal lobes control sensory information and proprioception.
- Hearing, olfaction, and short-term memory are controlled in two temporal lobes.
- Occipital lobe- visual cortex.

The limbic system is a collection of structures in the brain that control emotions and behavioral responses.

Blood-brain barrier- Selectively permeable, preserves homeostasis of the central nervous system.

Hypothalamus- connected to the pituitary gland. Regulated temperature, endocrine, water balance, carbohydrate, and fat metabolism. Affects the awake state and is a hormonal feedback system.

Brainstem- Respiratory control center. Provides messages to and from the cerebral structures to the spinal cord.

Cranial Nerves and functions

1. Olfactory- Smell
2. Optic- Vision
3. Oculomotor- Eye movement
4. Trochlear- Eye movement
5. Trigeminal- Allows sensation on the face, the face's skin, and the cornea's function.
6. Abducens- Eye movement
7. Facial- Taste on the anterior of the tongue
8. Acoustic auditory vestibulocochlear- Hearing and equilibrium
9. Glossopharyngeal- Taste on the posterior tongue, pharyngeal muscles
10. Vagus- Thoracic and abdominal organs, pharyngeal and laryngeal muscles.
11. Spinal accessory- Sternocleidomastoid and trapezius muscles
12. Hypoglossal- Tongue movement

Glossary of Neurology terms

- Choreiform movements- Rapid, jerky, purposeless movements made by multiple parts of the body.

- Brudzinski's sign- With passive flexion of the neck, the patient will demonstrate flexion of the hips and knees. This may help with diagnosing meningitis.

- Decerebrate posturing- Can be identified by rigid extension and adduction, and pronation of the arms and rigid extension and plantar flexion of the legs. The condition can be caused by severe injury to the brain and/or brain stem, resulting in overstimulation of the posture righting and the vestibular reflexes.

- Decorticate posturing- Flexion of the arms, wrist, and fingers with adduction of upper extremities with extension, internal rotation.
Believed to occur in patients with disruption of corticospinal pathways.

- Fasciculations- When the patient is in a resting state, fine twitching is noted. This can be normal in fatigue or in patients with lower motor neuron disorders such as polio, amyotrophic lateral sclerosis, or peripheral nerve disease.

- Kernig's sign- When the patient's leg is flexed at the hip and knee, the patient will experience resistance and pain. The hamstring is stiff and shows the inability to straighten the leg when the

162

hip is flexed. This may be done to help diagnose meningitis, which shows meningeal irritation.

- Monro-Kellie hypothesis- The skull is a ridged container that contains fixed volumes of contents. If one area is increased, another area must decrease. For example- an increase in blood volume will cause a decrease in the area of brain tissue, which will increase the ICP.

Intracranial pressure monitoring (ICP) –

A transducer may be connected to monitor to observe waveforms. The ICP waveform shows three peaks that are caused by vascular or arterial pulsations.

Normal measurement of ICP is less than 20 mm Hg. Changes in ICP measurements can occur before any clinical changes. Signs of increased ICP include:

- Confusion
- Restless
- Severe headache
- Nausea and projectile vomiting
- Visual field deficits
- Nuchal rigidity- Difficulty with flexing the neck

Later signs of increased ICP include:

- Decreased responsiveness.
- Change in level of consciousness.
- Changes in respiration- Irregular or apnea

Assessment of drainage from ear or surgical site for glucose- place liquid on white gauze. Cerebral spinal fluid will develop a ring.

163

Spinal cord injury- Patient needs to lay flat but may be turned to the side to promote airway and drainage of secretions.

Seizures:
- Focal or partial seizure- Involves unilateral neurons with a superficial focus. The patient may maintain consciousness if the seizure activity is limited to one hemisphere of the brain.
- Tonic-clonic/ generalized seizure- Bilateral neurons are affected. The seizure usually originates from a deeper brain focus. The patient will always lose consciousness with this type of seizure.

Procedures and surgery:

Craniotomy- Burr holes placed with the removal of a bone flap. Craniectomy is the removal of part of the skull without replacing it. Cranioplasty is the repair of skull defects.

- Infratentorial craniotomy- The patient needs to lie flat in bed. Flexion of the neck can cause sutures to tear. The patient can be placed on their side to promote away and drainage of oral secretions.

164

- Supratentorial craniotomy: Keep the patient's head off the bed at 30-45 degrees to decrease the chance of hemorrhage and promote venous drainage from the brain. The patient can turn to the side, but their neck needs to stay in alignment. Avoid placing the patient on the operative side after tumor removal to prevent increased ICP.

- Transsphenoidal surgery- Place the patient in high fowlers position to promote venous return from the brain to prevent increased ICP.

Blood patch- Patients can experience severe headaches after lumbar punctures and spinal anesthetics. A small amount of the patient's blood is injected into the area where the lumbar puncture was done to relieve the pain.

Burr hole- Removal of small circular sections of the skull for purposes of a craniotomy, drainage, or placement of monitoring equipment.

Carotid endarterectomy- May use a graft, anastomosis, or patch. Removal of plaque in vessels or can bypass occlusions. This procedure is discussed here due to the complication of stroke if the patient occludes the carotid. Neuro checks are a part of postoperative care for these patients.

Discectomy, microdiscectomy- Removal of disk or small fragments. Microdiscectomy has the advantage of decreasing infection risk, the ability to ambulate sooner, and decreasing the risk of CSF leakage.

Foraminotomy- The intervertebral foramen is enlarged to accommodate the exit of the spinal nerves.

Laminectomy- Decompression of the spinal cord or nerves. Spinal fusion may be performed at the same time.

Rhizotomy- Performed to interrupt the transmission of pain. Destroy the nerve root at the entrance of the spinal cord.

Spinal fusion- Insertion of bone chips between vertebrae. Hardware such as screws or bolts may be used. The procedure used for stabilization of the spinal column. If completed on the lumbar spine, the patient may have no limitation of movement. If completed on the cervical spine, the patient may have a limitation of movement. An anterior approach may be used.

Postoperative monitoring and care include:

- Bowel and bladder function,
- Log roll patient per surgeon instructions, and keep the patient in neutral alignment.
- Assess extremities for strength and sensation.
- Hematoma formation

Transsphenoidal hypophysectomy- Surgery on the pituitary gland through an incision inside the upper lip.

Postoperative assessments after neuro and spinal surgery and procedures-

- Headaches can indicate meningitis.
- Respiratory status may be affected depending on the type of surgery, such as the cervical spine.

- Monitor urinary status. Depending on the type of surgery or injury, such as lower spine, may affect the patient's ability to urinate.
- Monitor for leaking CSF.
- Hematomas
- New deficits in mobility or worsening of deficits.
- Autonomic dysreflexia
- Body alignment typically avoids twisting. Follow the surgeon's orders for specialized positioning.

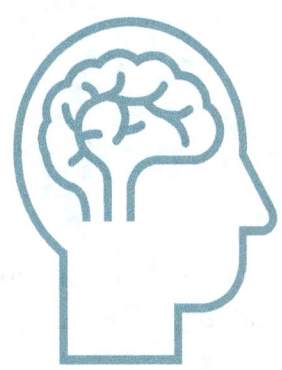

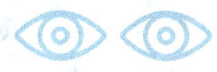

Ophthalmic Surgery

Anatomy:

Conjunctiva- Mucous membrane covering sclera and inner eyelid.

Lacrimal apparatus- Produces and drains tears.

Cornea- A window in which light rays pass.

Iris- Colored part of the eye that regulates the amount of light entering the eye. Divides space between the cornea and lens.

Retina- Receives images of objects and transfers them to the occipital lobe via the optic nerve.

Aqueous humor- Fluid that maintains ocular pressure.

Vitreous body- Gelatinous mass that supports the posterior cavity and keeps the retina in place.

Medications are commonly seen in eye surgery:

- Mydriatics- dilators- Phenylephrine-Block the accommodating ciliary muscle of the lens.

- Cycloplegics- dilators- Act on ciliary muscles

  o Atropine
  o Epinephrine
  o Tropicamide
  o Scopolamine

- BSS- irrigant that contains bicarbonate, dextrose, and glutathione.

- Steroids- Dexamethasone, prednisolone, and fluorometholone.

- Injectable anti-infective- Cefazolin, vancomycin, tobramycin.

- Cocaine- topical- Used on the cornea to loosen epithelium.

- Mitomycin- antimetabolite used to inhibit scar formation in Glaucoma. This is a chemotherapeutic drug; use caution.

- Miotics- Constrict the pupil.
  o Cholinergic
  o Anticholinesterase

- Osmotic agents- Lower intraocular pressure- Mannitol, glycerin

Ocular blocks:

The patient may be given IV sedation to help them relax for the procedure. The patient may need their eye taped closed after the procedure since they may not have a blink reflex.

Retrobulbar block- Causes loss of voluntary eye muscle control. The block is placed behind the eye to block the ciliary ganglion and nerves. Risks include brainstem anesthesia.

Peribulbar block- Less chance of hitting the optic nerve or causing brainstem anesthesia than the retrobulbar block. This block is given outside of the muscle cone.

Sub-Tenon block- A nasal incision is made. There is less chance of perforating the globe compared to other blocks. This block takes longer to take effect.

Dressings may include soft pads or taped to the patient or corneal shields placed on the eye.

Procedures:

Cataract surgery is one of the most common surgeries performed in ambulatory settings. Cataracts can be caused by genetics, trauma, infection, or chemical imbalances such as those caused by diabetes. Patient education includes:

- Do not rub the eye.
- Follow the doctor's instructions on the use of shields, eyeglasses, and dressings. The patient may need to tape the eye shield for bed at night.
- Sudden onset of pain or swelling should be reported to the doctor immediately.

Types:

- Extracapsular cataract extraction (ECCE)- Anterior portion of the capsule is removed after being ruptured, and the posterior capsule is left, which gives support to the new lens.

- Intracapsular cataract extraction (ICCE)- Removal of the lens, anterior and posterior capsule. This type has an increased risk of vitreous humor loss.

- Phacoemulsification- Ultrasonic vibrations fragment the lens, which is then aspirated. A small incision is needed.

Corneal transplant- The eye patch should remain in place until the surgeon says to remove it. Healing of the cornea is slow and may require repeated surgeries.

Types:

- Penetrating keratoplasty- Full thickness
- Lamellar keratoplasty- partial thickness, higher success rate than full thickness but more difficult.
- Keratectomy- Peeling of the cornea

Blepharoplasty- Repair of the eyelids. Iced saline dressings may be used postoperatively. The excess skin may impair the patient's vision, or the patient may want to improve their appearance.

Dacryocystorhinostomy (DCR)- The establishment of a new tear passageway that drains into the nasal cavity. A stent is placed that is usually removed in six weeks. The patient will need instructions on caring for the tube, how to sneeze, and how to put it back in if it falls out.

Ectropion- The patient's eyelid is turned outward, which may cause inflammation of the cornea. Bell's palsy, congenital issues may cause it or can be a normal aging condition.

Entropion- Caused by a spasm of the orbicularis oculi muscle. The patient's eyelashes turn in and scrape the cornea. This procedure removes excess skin. Cryotherapy may be used to freeze and remove lashes.

Glaucoma procedures-

- Iridectomy- Removal of a section of the iris for the treatment of acute, sub-acute, or chronic angle-closure glaucoma. This procedure re-establishes communication between the posterior and anterior chambers.
- Trabeculectomy- This procedure facilitates the drainage of aqueous humor from the posterior chamber to the anterior chamber.

Laser procedures- Lasers may be used in a variety of procedures. Lasers can be less invasive than other types of procedures. Types of lasers may include argon or yttrium aluminum garnet (YAG).

Ptosis- Drooping of the upper eyelid.

Retina surgery may cause pain for the patient. Orbital blocks and oral pain medication may be needed. Visual impairment postoperatively may cause emotional distress.

Post-operative positioning may be uncomfortable for the patient. Discuss the doctor's positioning requirements with the patient, such as the need to remain sitting. For retinopexy, for example, the patient will need to remain facedown for several days or weeks. This allows the bubble that was introduced to stay in place to allow the retinal tear or hole to heal.

Retinal detachment- The retina is separated from the choroid. Trauma, inflammatory processes, normal aging, or vascular disease may cause it. Signs and symptoms include loss of vision without pain, sudden onset of "Floaters," or a progressive slow decrease in the visual field. Educate the patient on the importance of following the surgeon's orders on physical limitations and the possibility of a long surgical time.

- Diathermy- No longer a common procedure. Microneedles deliver shortwave radio frequency energy. Causes scar formation with retinal reattachment at the area of adhesion.

- Cryotherapy- 80 degrees Celsius to the scleral area of detachment. The adhesions cause reattachment.

- Pneumoretinopexy- Injection of air or gases into the vitreous cavity. The patient will need to hold their head at a determined angle to allow healing.

- Laser- Welds retina into place.

- Scleral buckling- Creation of an indent in the retina so adherence can occur.

- Posterior vitrectomy- Removal of vitreous humor to allow the surgeon to work on the retina.

Strabismus- Inability to look at the same object with both eyes. This procedure to correct is commonly done on children. May see bradycardia with manipulation of the rectus muscle, treated with atropine.

Vitrectomy- Removal of the vitreous gel. It may be indicated for patients with advanced diabetic eye disease, trauma, or opacities. The procedure may take up to 6 hours. It may occur during cataract surgery. The patient may complain of severe pain. Pain medications and ice packs to the eye may help.

Pre- and post-operative care

The patient may be very anxious before surgery. No one wants a needle in their eye. Explanations on what to expect are appreciated. Common post-op instructions may include-

- Do not rub the eye.
- Avoid heavy lifting.
- Avoid activities that may increase intraocular pressure, such as vomiting or coughing.
- If sedation is given, encourage the patient to have someone with them for 24 hours, to not drink alcohol, or make any big decisions.
- Wear the eye shield or patch as ordered by the surgeon.
- May need to avoid reading if ordered.
- Do not drive until the surgeon allows it.

Oral/ Maxillofacial

Patients may come to the hospital for facial or dental surgery if they experience trauma, need a procedure that requires general anesthesia or have comorbidities that are too severe for the procedure to be completed at the dentist's office.

The patient may need to be nasally intubated.

Monitor for bleeding postoperatively; hemostasis may be difficult for some types of surgeries. The patient may have packing and monitor for aspiration.

Prepare to manage secretions and have suction available.

Pain control is important post-op. The surgeon may or may not want ice; ice may damage sensitive areas through vasoconstriction. Edema may be significant.

Nausea and vomiting may be present. The anesthetic used, low blood sugar levels from being NPO, and possibly blood in the stomach may cause nausea.

Instruct the patient on oral care post-op. Encourage the patient to use lubricant on lips if edematous for comfort. Avoid extremes of hot or cold food.

Orthopedic

Orthopedic surgeries often use tourniquets to create a less bloody surgical field. The surgeon is able to identify structures more easily with decreased bleeding. Nurses should use caution when placing tourniquets to help maintain skin integrity. The post-op nurse should assess the site to ensure the skin is not harmed. Prolonged tourniquet time may also cause nerve injury.

A cast may be placed to prevent the patient from moving the injured area. Plaster casts should be kept dry; use a plastic bag if going out in the rain or in the shower. If The cast is fiberglass, the surgeon may allow it to get wet and ask if there is a wound under the cast. Wounds inside a cast should not get wet. The patient may still have a cast that is drying when arriving at the recovery room. Fiberglass casts typically dry faster than plaster. Make sure there are no sharp edges that may damage the patient's skin. Assess the neuro status of the extremity for color movement sensation and temperature to ensure that the cast is not too tight.

Tell the patient not to put anything inside the cast, even if it itches. This could cause an infection. Teach the patient how to check the skin's color, movement, sensation, and temperature and call if the area becomes cold, numb, or shows signs of infection.

Typically, ice is placed on the extremity to help reduce swelling and pain. Elevate the extremity if allowed. For most ortho surgeries, neurovascular checks of the affected extremity are appropriate.

Traction may be applied for short-term immobilization of a fracture. Buck's traction is an example that is used for femoral fractures. Monitor the patient's skin to prevent pressure injuries.

Orthopedic patients are at high risk for DVT. Patients are often immobile and may be trauma victims and may not want to move due to pain. Monitor for signs and symptoms of DVT- edema that is not relieved with elevation, warmth, or redness.

A CPM- (continuous passive movement) machine may be used. Follow the surgeon's orders on settings and length of time used.

Medication that may be used:

- Bone wax- A mix of beeswax and isopropyl palmitate helps control bleeding.
- Topical thrombin- Reduce bleeding.

Anatomy:

Types of bone:

- Cortical (Compact)- Hard bone forming the outer shell. This type of bone is found in the shafts of long bones. Poor blood supply.
- Cancellous (Trabecular)- Soft and spongy. Contains red bone marrow. Found at the ends of long bones and in vertebrae. Has a rich blood supply.

Collagenous tissue- connective tissue derived from dense connective tissue.

- Tendons- attach muscle to bone.
- Ligaments- connect bone to bone.
- Fascia- Covers the muscles and provides nerves, blood, and lymph vessels.

Grafts may be used- Autografts- from the patient, allografts- from someone else. Autografts of cancellous may be taken from the ilium, olecranon, or distal radius. Cortical grafts may be taken from the tibia, fibula, iliac crest, or ribs.

Bone disorders and conditions

Compartment syndrome- A increased pressure in the muscle compartment. It can be caused by trauma or fracture. The pressure compromises nerves and vessels and can progress to ischemia. Permanent damage may occur. A fasciotomy may be required.

Fractures-

- **Avulsion**- A separation of a bone at the site of a ligament or tendon.

- **Colles fracture**- Fracture of the distal radius within one inch of the joint.
- **Compound/ open**- Involves an external wound.
- Incomplete- A green stick fracture is an example. The bone is not fractured all the way through.
- Impacted- Bone is driven into adjacent bone.
- **Pott's fracture**- Distal fibula fracture associated with tibiofibular disruption.
- **Spiral**

Disorders

Osteomyelitis- Acute or chronic infection of the bone.

Osteoporosis- Reduction in bone mass and strength results in a higher risk for fractures.

Paget's disease- Enlarged and deformed bones that may break down and weaken.

Rheumatoid arthritis- Autoimmune disorder potentially affecting multiple organs. Fibrinous pericarditis, pulmonary nodules, and bowel vasculitis are disorders that may be associated with rheumatoid arthritis.

Procedures:

ACL (Anterior Cruciate Ligament) repair- Improves joint stability in the knee. ACL is the most commonly torn or injured ligament. The ACL Contains receptor sites for estrogen, progesterone, and relaxin. Injuries are seen more often in female athletes- during menstruation, the estrogen causes ligaments to relax. Women also tend to have wider pelvises, which can cause a difference in stance to men, predisposing females to more injuries. The patient may receive a nerve block such as a femoral block for pain control.

Amputations- May be done for trauma, infection or vascular issues. Monitor for "Phantom pain".

Arthroplasty- Reconstruction or replacement of a joint. Procedure completed for patients with chronic pain or correction of a deformity. Postoperative monitoring includes neurovascular checks, wound care, and pain management. Drains may be placed. Postoperative Special care is needed with hip replacements- do not allow hip flexion greater than 90 degrees, hip adduction, or extremes in hip rotation.

Arthroscopy- Can be performed on multiple joints, such as the shoulder, wrist, knee, and ankle. Debridement, biopsy, repairs, and removal of loose bodies may be done arthroscopically.

Carpal tunnel release- The median nerve is decompressed by dividing the transverse carpal ligament. This patient typically receives MAC anesthesia care and may be fast-tracked to phase 2.

Closed reduction of fracture- The surgeon manipulates the fracture and may place a cast.

De Quervain's hand release-The dorsal compartment of the hand is decompressed to treat stenosing tenosynovitis of the wrist at the base of the thumb.

External fixation- a patient who has a severe wound or open fracture may need an external fixator placed. This allows fracture stabilization away from the site, lack of casting material, and the ability to perform future procedures. Monitor for signs and symptoms of infection.

Open reduction with internal fixation- The bone is repaired with pins, plates, and/or other implants. A cast or splint may be placed.

Rotator cuff repair- Can be done open or arthroscopically depending on the surgeon and the amount of damage. Postoperatively the patient may have a sling with a pillow support to keep the arm at the prescribed angle. The patient should be encouraged to follow instructions for therapy and to not over or underuse the arm. Contractures or further damage may result.

Synovectomy- All or part of the synovial lining of a joint is removed to stop the progression of rheumatic destruction of a joint.

Otorhinolaryngologic surgery

Ear, nose, and throat surgeries are included in this section.

Anatomy:

Tonsils- These are part of the lymphatic system and assist in filtering the lymph of bacteria and other foreign materials.

o Palatine- almond-shaped structures located on each side of the throat.
o Lingual- Located below the palatine tonsils at the base of the tongue.
o Pharyngeal- Located in the oral cavity in the upper rear wall. Begin as a larger size in children and shrink in size during puberty.

Pre-operative considerations- Do not clip hair unless absolutely necessary. Consult with the surgeon to determine if hair needs to be removed or if it can be taped out of the way. Use clippers, not a razor for shaving. Clipping hair can increase the risk of infection if there are cuts or nicks and can be upsetting to the patient.

If a patient wears hearing aids, consider allowing them to wear the aids in the operating room to allow the patient to communicate with the staff. Be careful with the patient's hearing aids! They are expensive and may not be covered by insurance!

Medications

- Local/topical anesthetics- Cocaine, benzocaine, lidocaine, tetracaine.
- Vasoconstrictors- epinephrine, neo-synephrine
- Topical antibiotics
- Topical antifungals
- Topical steroids.

Common post-operative education:

- May need to elevate the head to sleep.
- May have nasal packing, which can make swallowing difficult.
- Limit the Valsalva maneuver- coughing, bearing down, to limit tissue damage and bleeding.
- How to use a mustache dressing- A folded 2x2 secured under the nose to catch drips.
- Do not forcefully blow the nose. Sneeze with mouth open to prevent pressure.
- Avoid rapidly moving the head for some otologic procedures.
- Use a humidifier.
- Rinse mouth as ordered.

- Voice rest if ordered.
- Signs and symptoms of infection should be reported.
- Weird noises such as popping or crackling are normal.

Assess for facial nerve damage- check for symmetry:

- Smile
- Stick out the tongue.
- Wrinkle forehead
- Squeeze eyes shut.
- Pucker lips

Due to the dressings and possible packing used, hearing may be initially diminished.

Frequent swallowing may indicate bleeding. Blood in the stomach may cause nausea or vomiting.

Procedures on the ear

Facial nerve decompression- Indicated for Bell's palsy or edema that may cause nerve pressure. Protect the eye on the operative side from corneal dryness. An incision is made of the facial nerve sheath at the area of compromise. A trans mastoid, trans labyrinthine, or middle cranial fossa approach may be used. The patient may require an ICU stay if a middle fossa approach is used.

Labyrinthectomy- Surgical destruction of the membranous labyrinth of the horizontal semicircular canal. The procedure is indicated for patients experiencing vertigo. Move the patient slowly in all phases of care to help prevent vertigo. Nausea and vomiting may be an issue for these patients. Assess the facial nerve. Taste changes may occur but will be temporary. Potential complications include CSF leaks, facial nerve paralysis, tinnitus, and meningitis.

Mastoidectomy- This can be simple, modified, or radical. Indicated for patients with acute or chronic infections or extension of cholesteatoma into mastoid cells. Elevate the patient's head to minimize edema, and lay the patient with the operative ear up to prevent pressure according to the surgeon's orders. Assess facial nerve function.

Myringotomy- A small incision is made into the posteroinferior aspect of the tympanic membrane to allow pressure relief and to place a tympanostomy tube if needed. This procedure may be done for patients who experience multiple infections with otitis media. The patients are often children. Discharge instructions include avoiding getting the ears wet, changing the cotton balls in the ears as directed, and that the tubes may fall out on their own.

Stapedectomy- To restore stapes bone function by removal of diseased stapes and replacing them with a prosthesis. Stiffening and hardening of the stapes can be caused by the formation of spongey bone around the round window. Elevate the patient's head to minimize edema, and lay the patient with the operative ear up to prevent graft displacement according to the surgeon's orders.

Tympanoplasty- Reconstructive surgery performed on the middle ear components to improve hearing and/or to prevent recurrent infection. May be performed in stages. Grafts such as cartilage, bone, skin, or other materials may be used. Assess facial nerve.

Procedures on the nose

Standard post-op care includes changing dressing when needed, encouraging the patient not to blow the nose, bend or strain, and sneeze with the mouth open. Swallowed blood may cause nausea and vomiting or bloody or black stools. If splints are left in place, the patient should not disturb.

Ethmoidectomy- The ethmoid is a pair of paranasal sinuses. The procedure is performed for the promotion of drainage. Ethmoid surgery or surgery near the area may cause orbital bruising.

Rhinoplasty- Repair of the nasal cartilage or fracture of the nose. It may be performed to improve cosmetic appearance. The patient may experience swelling for longer than they anticipated, which may cause anxiety.

Septoplasty- Restoration of the septum to repair intranasal and septal defects. The procedure may include the excision of cartilage or bone, a reduction of turbinate size (turbinectomy), or other procedures that improve defects that interfere with respiratory function. The patient may have splints or packing post-op. A mustache dressing may be in place. Frequent swallowing may indicate bleeding.

Sinus surgery- May be performed for diseased tissue to increase airflow. Monitor for possible complications such as CFS leak post-op.

Surgery on the throat and neck

Adenoidectomy and/ or tonsillectomy- May be performed at the same time. More common in the pediatric population. Encourage the patient to avoid clearing the throat, rest the voice, and eat a bland, soft diet. The patient should be told the pain may increase between post-op days 4 to 8 because of the "scab falling off." Frequent swallowing may indicate bleeding. Bleeding in the stomach may cause nausea, vomiting, or black or bloody stools.

Laryngectomy- Removal of the larynx. It may be partial or total. Commonly performed as a cancer treatment.

Laryngoscopy- Visualization of the larynx. A biopsy may be performed. Instruct the patient to rest their voice postoperatively. Monitor for laryngospasm.

Neck dissection- May be modified or radical. Commonly performed for cancer.

Phono surgery- Procedure performed to improve vocal cord mobility and to improve voice quality. A prosthesis may be inserted to maintain the vocal cord position- Silastic shim.

Salivary gland surgery- This may be parotidectomy or submandibular gland excision. Monitor for facial nerve damage.

- o Frey's syndrome- Occurs when the patient eats, sees, or thinks about food. The patient may sweat or flush in the cheek area.

Thyroidectomy- May include removal of the parathyroid gland. Elevate the head of the bed, have a tracheostomy kit available, and encourage deep breathing. Monitor for low calcium levels- cramping, numb lips. Monitor for thyroid storm- tachycardia, hypertension, heat intolerance, sweating.

Tracheostomy- Creating an artificial opening in the trachea. Keep all supplies at the bedside, such as the obturator or any ventilator connections. Elevate the head of the bed, and make sure trach ties are secure but not too tight. The patient may wish to communicate with pen and paper.

Podiatry

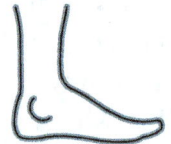

Anatomy-

Calcaneus- the big heel bone.

Metatarsals- five bones

Phalanges- Toes

Plantar- The sole of the foot

Disorders-

Corn- Thickening of the skin can cause irritation.

Hallux valgus- Bunion. A deformity of the first metatarsal and the great toe.

Mallet toe- Abnormality of the distal interphalangeal joint. It may be congenital, caused by pressure on the toes from shoes. Most commonly, the second toe.

Post-op care may include crutches and a surgical boot. The patient may be allowed to walk or may have restrictions.

If a patient is sent home with a cast, remind the patient not to stick anything inside the cast, even if it itches. This is a great way to get an infection. The patient may need to put the cast in a plastic bag to avoid getting wet when bathing.

Respiratory, Thoracic, and the Lungs

Assessment of breathing

- Cheyne-Stokes- Shallow to deeper, then shallow again breathing.

- Biot's- Regular or irregular periods of apnea followed by quick, shallow inspiration. This type of breathing may be caused by stroke or head trauma.

- Patients with COPD may demonstrate prolonged expiratory time.

- Fremitus- Vibrations felt through the chest wall.

- Anemia may cause false low oxygen saturation readings.

- Carboxyhemoglobinemia may cause false high oxygen saturation readings.

.

Stir-up regimen-
Stimulation, verbal
and tactile, to
encourage respiration

Anatomy

- There are 12 pairs of ribs.

- The thorax is an airtight space that receives air from the nasal passages, trachea, and bronchi.

- Inspiration takes place when the intrathoracic pressure is below the atmospheric pressure.

Respiratory Conditions

OSA-

Obstructive Sleep Apnea. Airway obstruction during sleep is due to reduced muscle tone in the airway.

- Higher incidence in obese patients.
- Increases risk for post-op complications.
- Occurs in 1-5% of the general population.

Testing For OSA:

194

- A sleep study or polysomnography- is considered the gold standard for OSA testing. This test can be expensive and requires the patient to spend the night hooked up to machinery in a lab.

- Berlin Questionnaire- The patient answers questions to help determine the risk of OSA.

- STOP-BANG- Acronym for:

  - Snore
  - Tired
  - Observed- patient's family has observed apnea while sleeping.
  - Pressure- Is the patient's blood pressure high?
  - Body mass index- over 35?
  - Age- Over 50?
  - Neck size- 16 inches or larger?
  - Gender- Male?

OSA care considerations:

- The patient may have more frequent desaturations.

- The patient may require extended monitoring.

- Positioning- avoid supine if possible. Sitting or lateral preferred.

- Consider using noninvasive positive pressure ventilation or CPAP.

  - CPAP- Delivers PEEP, delivers constant pressure.

- o BiPAP- Delivers PEEP, pressure support, and timed breaths. Reacts to changes in breathing. Non-invasive equivalent to a ventilator.

- Consider multimodal medications and treatments for pain, such as nerve blocks, or non-pharmaceuticals, such as ice.

- If on a PCA, basal is not recommended.

- Facility policy may require patients with OSA to be monitored longer. For example, a patient with OSA may be required to stay in recovery 4 hours after the last anesthesia medication before discharge home.

Laryngospasm-

Spasm of the larynx. Suctioning the airway before Extubation may prevent laryngospasm.

S/S:

- The patient's airflow is affected. Stridor, crowing, or absent breath sounds may be noted.
- Anxiety, panic
- Hypoxemia, hypercarbia

Treatment:

- Humidified O2, positive pressure ventilation
- Succinylcholine, steroids
- Reintubate

Bronchospasm-

It can be caused by an allergic response, aspiration, Histamine release, COPD, suctioning, and intubation.

S/S:

- Use of accessory muscles
- Decreased oxygen saturation.
- Tachypnea

Treatment

- Bronchodilator, muscle relaxant, lidocaine and epinephrine if severe
- Humidified oxygen

Atelectasis-

It can be caused by bronchial obstruction, decreased lung volume, decreased cardiac output, hypotension, and secretions.

S/S-

- Hypoxia
- Decreased breath sounds.
- Consolidation on chest X-ray

Treatment-

- Deep breathing
- Humidified oxygen
- Increased mobility
- Intermittent positive pressure breathing

- Confirm placement of ET if intubated.

Aspiration-

A foreign body or gastric contents can cause it. Common S/S include dyspnea, cyanosis, tachycardia, and cough. If gastric contents are aspirated- bronchospasm, hypoxemia, and atelectasis are common.

Pulmonary edema- Causes:

- Aspiration
- Disseminated intervascular coagulation (DIC
- Increased altitude
- Anaphylaxis
- Naloxone in young adults
- Sepsis
- Ischemic heart disease
- Laryngospasm
- Fluid overload
- Left ventricular failure.
- Mitral valve dysfunction

S/S

- Confusion
- Decreased lung compliance.
- Dyspnea
- Hypotension
- Hypoxemia
- Frothy pink sputum
- Jugular venous distention
- Pulmonary infiltrates on chest X-ray

- Tachycardia
- Tachypnea
- Wheezing

Treatment-

- Diuretics
- Afterload reduction
- Fluid restriction
- Reduce cardiac workload.
- Place the patient in an upright position.

Pulmonary treatments and interventions

Pain control for pulmonary procedures-

- Epidural
- Intrathecal opioid
- paravertebral analgesia- a catheter is placed in the paravertebral space for medication administration,
- extra pleural analgesia- via a space in the chest wall
- Intercostal nerve block
- Cryoanalgesia- Long-lasting intercostal nerve block

Bronchoscopy- Procedure to visualize the airway. Performed for conditions such as cancer, foreign bodies, abnormal tissues, and lavage. It may cause bronchospasm or laryngeal spasm.

Chest tube- Placed for complications such as pneumothorax, cardiac tamponade, empyema, pleural effusions, and others. The placement of the tube depends on the condition.

The chest drainage system may have a water seal that prevents the air from reentering the chest space. The chest tube may drain via wall suction, positive expiratory pressure, or gravity. When working properly, the system may produce a bubbling sound, but some types do not.

Check for subcutaneous emphysema or crepitus, a popping feeling in the chest with palpation. Subcutaneous emphysema may indicate an improperly placed chest tube.

Place a sterile dressing over the site if a chest tube is accidentally removed. A petroleum-impregnated dressing or other occlusive dressing is preferred. The idea is to allow air to escape but not go back in. An EMT told me once to use an unopened 4x4 gauze taped on one side. It would flap in the breeze as the patient took a breath and exhaled.

Decortication- Performed to improve lung function by removing fibrous tissue, cancer, or membranes on the visceral side and partial pleura.

Drainage of empyema- Empyema may be acute or chronic. It may require decortication. It may be associated with an infection.

Lobectomy- Removal of one or more lobes of the ling.

Lung volume reduction surgery- Performed on patients with emphysema to increase expiratory airflow, muscle strength, and exercise capacity.

Mediastinoscopy- A small incision is made above the suprasternal notch. Performed for biopsy of tumors or lymph nodes. It may cause pneumothorax, subcutaneous emphysema, or air embolism.

Pneumonectomy- Removal of the lung. Large lung tumors may need to be removed via clamshell or hemi-clamshell. The patient is positioned laterally in the operating room. The procedure is performed through the4tth and 5th intercostal space or maybe axillary.

VATS procedure- Video-assisted thoracoscopic surgery. Used for diagnosis, biopsy, wedge resections, lobectomy, or other procedures. It may be used in combination with robotic surgery.

RATS- Robotic-assisted thoracoscopic surgery- smaller incisions can help lower morbidity and have better pain control postoperatively.

The patient may come to the recovery room with an arterial line in place.

Fluid may be restricted due to the potential for ARDS- Acute Respiratory Distress Syndrome. For blood pressure control, Vaso-pressers are usually preferred. Potential complications include cardiac arrhythmias such as AFIB and diaphragm, liver, or spleen injury.

Thoracoscopy- Pleural cavity visualization to perform procedures such as decortication of hemothorax, biopsy, vagotomies, and others. Decortication is a procedure that removes fibrous tissue and pus from the pleural space.

Open window thoracoscopy involves resection of the ribs to allow for drainage and removal of empyema.

Thoracotomy- Incision in the chest wall to operate on the lungs.

Ventilator support

The intubated patient may be placed on a ventilator in the phase 1 recovery room for temporary care or for prolonged care if the PACU is used for an ICU overflow. Each ventilator is slightly different but provides ventilation assistance to patients. Some settings provide a defined amount of tidal volume to the patient, others PEEP, Some settings allow the patient to initiate breathing, and others automatically give the patient a breath.

Wedge resection- Removal of a wedge-shaped section of the parenchyma. Procedure performed for patients with identifiable lesions, chronic lung disease, and biopsy.

Medications-

- Picibanil- Treatment of pneumothorax.
- Talc- Used to treat spontaneous pneumothorax.

Vascular

Pre-operative considerations: Patients may lose large amounts of blood during vascular surgery. Remember that some patients do not want to receive blood products. A discussion may be necessary to explain the possible need for a transfusion and any devices, such as a cell saver, allowing the patient's blood to be infused.

Anatomy

- The three layers of arteries and veins-

    o Tunica intima- Inner layer
    o Tunica media- Middle layer, muscular layer. If an artery is severed, this muscular section may contract and constrict to help stop hemorrhage.
    o Tunica adventitia- Fibrous outer layer

- The autonomic nervous system regulates arteries and veins.

- The exchange of waste and nutrients is done at the capillary level.
- The term laminar refers to the movement of blood in parallel lines. If blood flow is disrupted, this is termed turbulence. Turbulence causes a bruit which can be auscultated or heard with a Doppler.

Medications

- Dopamine- A vasopressor that directly stimulates beta receptors and dopamine receptors. Low doses may be used to stimulate urine output by causing mesenteric and renal vasodilation.

- Esmolol (Brevibloc)- Beta blocker used to treat supraventricular tachyarrhythmias. It may cause hypotension.

- Heparin- anticoagulant

- Labetalol- Treatment for hypertension.

- Milrinone (Primacor)- Use with care- may cause thrombocytopenia. A positive inotropic agent that causes vasodilation.

- Nifedipine (Procardia)- Calcium channel blocker used to treat hypertension. Augments cardiac output and decreases systemic vascular resistance.

- Nitroglycerin- A vasodilator that relaxes smooth muscles in small blood vessels. Increased cardiac perfusion.

- Papaverine- Smooth muscle relaxant.

- Phenylephrine (Neo-Synephrine)- Vasoconstrictor causes increased peripheral resistance. Increases blood pressure. Acts on alpha-adrenergic receptors.

- Protamine- Anti-heparin agent

- Sodium nitroprusside (Nipride)- Vasodilator. Used to treat hypertension, reduces vascular resistance, and increase cardiac output.

Diseases and conditions

Acute or chronic arterial insufficiency- Can be caused by occlusion. Arteriosclerotic plaque may break loose, or a blood clot may be caused by arterial fibrillation or a myocardial infarct. Insufficiency may be acute or chronic. Chronic conditions may be caused by the build-up of calcium and cholesterol within the artery's wall. Ischemia can be a result of insufficiency.

Acute or chronic venous insufficiency- Acute venous insufficiency can be caused by deep vein thrombosis. Incompetent valves can cause chronic venous insufficiency. Chronic insufficiency can present with venous stasis ulcers. Pressure stockings may be used to help control chronic insufficiency. Duplex ultrasonography may be used to help with diagnosis.

Aneurysm- A true aneurysm is the dilation of all layers of the artery. A dissecting aneurysm results from a tear in the artery wall. A false aneurysm is a disruption through all the layers with escaping blood. Abdominal aortic aneurysms account for most aneurysms.

Cerebral vascular accident- May be caused by debris or clot which may occlude the vessels or a vessel rupture. It may be a TIA, an episode of brain dysfunction that resolves within 24 hours.

DVT- Deep vein thrombosis- Commonly caused by an intraluminal clot. If the clot becomes dislodged, it may travel to the lungs, causing a pulmonary embolism.

o   Virchow's triad- Hypercoagulability, venous stasis, intimal damage caused by ischemia or trauma.

Monckeberg's arteriosclerosis- Peripheral arteries are affected by calcium deposits within the medial layer.

Polyarthritis nodosa (PAN)- a systemic disease that causes arterial inflammation and possible aneurysm rupture. Kawasaki is a similar disease but occurs in children. Behcet's disease is similar but affects both arteries and veins.

Raynaud's- Vasospastic disease. It may be exacerbated by exposure to cold. It may have ischemic changes. The patient may experience numbness, cyanosis, and tingling.

Procedures

Post-operative considerations for all vascular may include monitoring for bleeding, pulses, pain, and swelling. Vascular surgeries may take a long time. Assess the patient skin for signs of pressure injury.

Patients should be monitored for perfusion at the operative site, neurologic condition, and CMST (Color, movement, sensation, temp) of the affected limb. The patient may be on vasoactive IV drips post-op. The patient may need invasive hemodynamic monitoring, including an arterial line or a Swan-Ganz catheter. Monitor the patient for EKG rhythm changes. The patient may come to the PACU intubated on a ventilator.

Bradycardia may be caused by vagal stimulation from manipulation or hematomas, altered baroreceptor responses, or MI.

A Doppler may be used pre- and post-op for assessments. A Doppler uses an ultrasound beam that is reflected back to the probe by moving red blood cells. An audible noise is created that sounds like "swish, swish." Some dopplers can be sterilized and used in the operating room.

Ankle Brachial Index or ankle arm index-ABI or AAI- Noninvasive test used to help diagnose peripheral artery disease.

Obtain the blood pressure of both arms and both legs. To determine the ABI for the right leg, divide the pressure from the leg by the highest pressure obtained from the arms. Normal is 1.0 to 1.4. 1.4 and above may suggest a calcified vessel and values below 0.9 may indicate peripheral arterial disease.

AAA- Abdominal aortic aneurysm. These typically occur between the renal arteries and the aortic bifurcation. AAA is usually asymptomatic and is found during routine exams. Dissection and rupture can cause hemorrhage and shock. A sudden tear in the aortic intima is a path for blood to enter the aortic wall. Post-operative considerations may include keeping the patient on a ventilator, invasive hemodynamic monitoring, and NG with NPO until bowel tones return.

An endovascular repair can be less invasive with the introduction of the endograft or stent through a femoral artery instead of abdominally. Morbidity, pain, and time of recovery are often reduced.

For all types of AAA repair, post-op care includes monitoring pulses in extremities and monitoring kidney function and pain. Back pain may be a symptom of AAA. Post-op education for the patient includes not lifting more than 5 pounds, driving until the doctor clears, and no tub baths, but showers are allowed.

Amputation- Limbs may need to be amputated for many reasons. The patient may experience negative emotions related to the loss of a limb. Phantom pain is a possible complication. The surgeon may use a tourniquet during surgery and check for skin integrity post-op.

- o Syme amputation is done through the ankle. A midcalf amputation is preferred due to

208

improved rehabilitation and possible prosthetics.

Arteriovenous fistula- Connects an artery and vein for long-term renal dialysis. Grafts may be used. Some examples include the radial artery to a cephalic vein, the ulnar artery to the basilic vein, or the brachial artery to a basilic or cephalic vein.

Some types of fistulas need to mature, which may take several weeks; others may be used immediately. Fistulas may have variable flow rates depending on the type. Avoid using the affected arm for blood pressure, lab draws, or any procedures that may affect the blood flow to the site. Palpate for a thrill, auscultate for bruit. Monitor dressings to ensure there is no tight, circumferential pressure. The patient may be ordered to keep the limb elevated, avoid tight clothing, and be taught how to palpate thrill.

o Steal syndrome- ischemia related to vascular inefficiency. Look for diminished pulses, pain, and pallor. Surgery to the site may be needed to repair.

Bypass- Anastomosis or graft to divert blood flow from an area of low blood flow due to disease or clot to improve blood flow. It may be done around the occlusion. Examples are femoral to femoral, femoral to popliteal, or axillofemoral.

Carotid endarterectomy- Removal of an atheroma- atherosclerotic plaque. This procedure is done to increase cerebral perfusion. A shunt may be inserted. Be aware the patient may experience reperfusion headaches. Numbness that reaches the ear is common. Teach the patient's family to watch for mental status changes. Monitor for hypotension, hypertension, and cerebral artery perfusion. The patient may be on vasoactive IV medications post-op.

Femoropopliteal and femorotibial bypass- Grafts are used to bypass occluded sections of the artery. The graft may be synthetic or a saphenous vein.

Percutaneous transluminal angioplasty- Used to treat short-segment occlusions. In a minimally invasive procedure, local anesthetic is used, and it may be a same-day procedure.

Vein stripping and excision- Treatment for varicose veins. In pre-op, the patient may stand so the surgeon can mark the legs for the surgical site.

Vena cava filter- A filter such as a greenfield filter is placed in the vena cava to maintain patency by trapping emboli. Typically placed through the right groin.

Post-operative teaching includes instructing the patient not to bend the operative leg for eight hours, avoid strenuous activity, elevate the leg, and use elastic stockings to help reduce swelling. The patient may be prescribed DVT prophylaxis.

Varicose vein surgery- Educate the patient that sitting and standing in one place should be limited.

The six Ps of neurovascular assessment

Pulses

Pain

Paresthesia

Paralysis

Pallor

Poikilothermic- Cold

Recommended Reading and References

The following are recommended readings for further knowledge and to help study for certification exams. I recommend you try and find the most recent edition.

Cpancapa.org. *Certification Candidate Handbook.*

American Society of PeriAnesthesia Nurses (2019-2020). *Perianesthesia Nursing*

ASPAN. *Standards Practice Recommendations and Interpretive Statements.* New Jersey,

American Heart Association. *ACLS Provider Manual.* Use the most current edition.

American Heart Association. *PALS Provider Manual.* Use the most current edition.

Chatterjee, K. (2009) The Swan-Ganze Catheters: Past, Present, and Future, *Circulation, 119*(1).

Malignant Hyperthermia Association of the United States, www.mhaus.org

Marsh, T. (2021). *The Certified Ambulatory Perianesthesia Nurse CAPA Study Guide.*

Marsh, T. (2021). *Certified Post-anesthesia Nurse CPAN Study Guide.*

Odom-Forren, J. (2018). *Drain's Perianesthesia Nursing, A Critical Care Approach.* St. Louis, Missouri, Elsevier.

Rothrock, J. (2019). *Alexanders Care of the Patient in Surgery sixteenth edition.* St. Louis, Missouri, Elsevier.

Schick, L., Windle, P. (2021). *Perianesthesia Nursing Core Curriculum: Preprocedure, Phase 1 and Phase 2 PACU Nursing.* St. Louis, Missouri, Elsevier.

Vallerand, A. & Sanoski, C. (2021). *Davis's Drug Guide for Nurses seventeenth Edition,* F.A. Davis Company, Philadelphia, PA.

CPAN Practice Questions

1) Which category would a patient with a ruptured abdominal aortic aneurysm be placed?

   A) ASA 6

   B) ASA 5

   C) ASA 4

   D) ASA 3

2) Which of the following would a sphenopalatine block be appropriate?

   A) Back pain

   B) Pelvic pain

   C) Chest pain

   D) Chronic headaches

3) A positive Chvostek's sign indicates which of the following?

   A) Calcium deficiency

   B) Sodium deficiency

   C) Potassium deficiency

   D) Potassium excess

4) Pain in the calf when the foot is flexed in the presence of a possible blood clot is called:

   A) Trousseau's sign

   B) Homan's sign

   C) Babinski sign

   D) Palmer's sign

5) The inability to shrug a shoulder would indicate damage to which cranial nerve?

   A) Abducens

   B) Glossopharyngeal

   C) Spinal accessory

   D) Vagus

6) A patient comes to the PACU after a pneumonectomy on the right side. How should you not position the patient?

A) On the right side

B) On the left side

C) Semi fowlers

D) Supine

7) After an assessment of the phase 1 PACU, it has been determined that the nurses are suffering from alarm fatigue. Which of the following is not a recommendation to combat alarm fatigue?

A) Deactivate all alarms.

B) Develop a process that identifies which alarms can be deactivated.

C) Adjust alarms to the individual patient's needs.

D) Educate nurses on the use of the device.

8) A patient's heart condition causes cardiac insufficiency with persistent angina and dysrhythmia. Which of the following classifications does this patient belong?

A) ASA 7

B) ASA 6

C) ASA 5

D) ASA 4

9) You are assisting the anesthesiologist in the operating room before your patient's surgery. The patient is given an anesthetic. The anesthesiologist tests the patient's eyelid reflex with no response. You note the patient has irregular respirations. What stage of anesthesia is the patient in?

A) Stage 1

B) Stage 2

C) Stage 3

D) Stage 4

10) Your patient received an infratentorial craniotomy. What position should the patient be placed in?

A) Flat, turned to the side to provide an adequate airway.

B) High fowlers

C) Head of bed 30 to 40 degrees

D) Prone

CPAN Practice Questions Answers and Rationale

1) B

A moribund patient who is not expected to survive without surgery is given a classification of ASA 5. Multisystem trauma would also fall into this category.

2) D

A sphenopalatine block would be appropriate for chronic headaches.

3) A

Chvostek's sign is an abnormal spasm in the face when the face is tapped at the angle of the jaw. This can indicate a deficiency in calcium.

4) B

Homan's sign is a pain in the leg, most commonly in the calf when the foot is dorsiflexed.

5) C

The spinal accessory nerve controls the sternocleidomastoid and trapezius muscles. The inability to move a shoulder may indicate damage to this nerve. Damage to the abducens nerve may be a medial deviation of the eye. Loss of the gag reflex may indicate damage to the glossopharyngeal nerve. Similar symptoms may be present with damage to the vagus nerve, with the inclusion of the patient experiencing a hoarse voice.

6) B

Do not place the patient on the non-operative side.
Place the patient on the operative side to help increase
lung expansion.

7) A

It recommended NOT to deactivate all alarms. All other
choices are recommendations to decrease alarm fatigue.

8) D

ASA 7 is not a classification. ASA 6 is a brain-dead
patient. ASA 5 is a patient who will die without
surgery; this is not indicated in the question. ASA 4 is a
patient with a severe systemic disease that is a constant
threat to life.

9) B

The patient is in the stage of delirium, which is stage 2.
The patient is at risk in this stage for laryngospasm,
cardiac arrest, and vomiting.

10) A

The patient who has received an infratentorial
craniotomy should be flat. A patient who has received a
transsphenoidal surgery should have the head of the bed
in a high fowlers position. A patient who has received a
supratentorial craniotomy should have the head of the
bed at 30 to 45 degrees. Most patients should not be
prone.

CAPA Practice Questions

1) Which of the following is true?

   A) All patients have a right to information about treatment.

   B) A patient who has a mental health diagnosis is incapable of making an informed decision about their own healthcare.

   C) A patient may make an informed care decision regardless of if the risks and benefits are explained.

   D) The patient can be enrolled in a research study without consent if the knowledge of being in the study would be contraindicated to the study.

2) A six-year-old is admitted with acute appendicitis. The patient has varicella- chicken pox. Which of the following is the correct action?

A) Place the patient in contact precautions.

B) Place the patient in a negative pressure room.

C) Place the patient in a positive pressure room.

D) Do nothing since chicken pox is not contagious to adults.

3) Which of the following is correct in regard to the elderly patient and medication?

A) Decrease in serum concentration of water-soluble drugs.

B) The decreased half-life of fat-soluble drugs

C) A decrease in the accumulation of drugs

D) Decrease in the rate of drug clearance by the liver.

4) Aspirin can affect platelet adhesives for how long for most patients?

A) 2 days

B) 3 days

C) 7 days

D) 2 weeks

5) Your patient arrives in the PACU after a laparoscopic procedure that was converted to open cholecystectomy. You take the first set of vital signs and note that the patient is hypertensive. Which of the following may be the cause?

A) The patient is hypovolemic

B) The patient's blood pressure cuff is too large

C) The patient's blood pressure cuff is too small

D) The patient recently received phenylephrine.

6) Which of the following are safe for a patient with a Family history of malignant hyperthermia?

A) Nitrous oxide

B) Halothane

C) Sevoflurane

D) Succinylcholine

7) Which of the following anesthetic agents would be avoided for patients having surgery on the middle ear?

A) Desflurane

B) Nitrous oxide

C) Isoflurane

D) Sevoflurane

8) Your patient is having a scleral buckle today. You know the patient understands the procedure when they say:

A) I am having the gel inside of my eye removed.

B) I am having a piece of silicone sewn into my eye to correct my retinal detachment.

C) I am having my rotator cuff repaired.

D) I am having my cataract removed

9) Your patient is scheduled for a goniotomy. You know this procedure is performed for patients with which condition?

A) Retinal tear

B) Congenital conditions of the testes

C) Tumor in the frontal lobe

D) Glaucoma

10) A surgeon wants to add a case for later today to repair a hip fracture for a patient admitted during the night. You call and get the report and learn the patient ate breakfast at 0600 with eggs, bacon, and milk. What time is the earliest the patient can have surgery?

A) The patient cannot have surgery today.

B) 1000

C) 1400

D) 1800

CAPA Practice Questions Answers and Rationale

1) A

   All patients have a right to information about their treatment and are given the ability to make treatment decisions unless the patient is determined incapable by law. A mental health diagnosis does not automatically remove the rights of the patient. All research subjects have the right to make an informed decision about participating in a study.

2) B

   Patients with chickenpox should be placed in airborne precautions, including a negative pressure room. Unfortunately, adults can contract chickenpox.

3) D

   In the elderly, a decrease in the rate of drug clearance by the liver is commonly seen. The accumulation of drugs increases in the elderly. The half-life of fat-soluble drugs and the serum concentration of water-soluble drugs is not decreased in the elderly.

4) C

Aspirin usually affects platelet adhesiveness for seven days in most people.

5) C

Blood pressure may be inaccurate if the blood pressure cuff is not the correct size. A too-small cuff may give the patient an incorrectly high reading. The other choices may cause hypotension.

6) A

Of the medications listed, only nitrous oxide is safe for a patient with a family history of malignant hyperthermia

7) B

Nitrous oxide is more soluble than nitrogen which may cause enclosed gas-filled spaces in the body to expand. Surgery involving the middle ear, intestinal obstructions, and pneumothorax typically will not use nitrous oxide.

8) B

A scleral buckle is the correction of a retinal detachment. Vitrectomy is the removal of the vitreous gel to clear blood occluding vision. Removal of a cataract would include phacoemulsification.

9) D

A goniotomy is a procedure for congenital glaucoma.

10) C

It is common practice for surgery to be delayed 6 to 8 hours after a patient has eaten a full meal.

www.ingramcontent.com/pod-product-compliance
Lightning Source LLC
Chambersburg PA
CBHW082209290526
45794CB00009B/3480